Surgery of the Heart

The Coventry Conference

Surgery of the Heart

The Coventry Conference

EDITED BY

J. A. Dyde

Walsgrave Hospital
Coventry, England

AND

R. E. Smith

Warwickshire Postgraduate Medical Centre
Coventry, England

Plenum Medical Book Company ● New York and London

Library of Congress Cataloging in Publication Data

Main entry under title:

Surgery of the heart.

"Proceedings of a conference organized by the Warwickshire Postgraduate Medical
Centre held in Coventry, England, September 11-12, 1975.
Includes index.
1. Heart—Surgery—Congresses. I. Dyde, J. A. II. Smith, Ronald Edward. III. War-
wickshire Postgraduate Medical Centre. [DNLM: 1. Heart surgery—Congresses.
WG168 S964 1975]
RD598.S85   617'.412   76-14827
ISBN-13: 978-1-4613-4285-4   e-ISBN-13: 978-1-4613-4283-0
DOI: 10.1007/978-1-4613-4283-0

Proceedings of a Conference organized by the Warwickshire
Postgraduate Medical Centre held in Coventry, England,
September 11-12, 1975

©1976 Plenum Publishing Corporation
227 West 17th Street, New York, N. Y. 10011
Softcover reprint of the hardcover 1st edition 1976

Plenum Medical Book Company is an imprint of Plenum Publishing Corporation

PREFACE

DR. R. E. SMITH

The first and second Coventry conferences on "Surgery of the Oesophagus" and "Surgery of the Lung" were arranged by Mr. Roger Abbey Smith, and they were so successful that he asked his colleague, Mr. J. A. Dyde to arrange one on "Surgery of the Heart." He willingly accepted this task and has also been joint Editor. This book reproduces as faithfully as possible the papers and the discussion on the various subjects included in the Coventry conference.

The simple title "Surgery of the Heart" could be expanded to include the blood vessels. Especially important is the anatomy of the various combinations and permutations of the pulmonary and systemic vessels. These play a major role in the production of pulmonary hypertension. First class investigations by radiologists, and physiologists ascertain the precise situation which the surgeon will expect to find when he opens the chest; indeed will help him to make the right approach.

Mr. W. G. Williams helped with the social programme which enabled people to meet people. Mr. A. Martin gave us valuable help in taping the recordings which Mrs. J. Jelley and Mrs. V. Bayliss-Stranks ably transcribed. The editorial staff of Plenum Publications have given us unsparing advice and guidance.

PROLOGUE

DR. R. E. SMITH

I welcome you all to this conference on Surgery of the Heart.
It is the third conference we have had on surgery of the thorax,
and some are here for the first time, some for the second, and a
few for the third.

Many people are enjoying longer and happier lives thanks to
knowledge engendered by Physicians, Surgeons, Anaesthetists,
Physiologists, Radiologists, Nurses and Technicians, and it is
a pleasure to see all those disciplines represented here.

Coventry has maintained its long interest in cardiology. A
landmark was in 1946, when Captain G. T. Smith Clarke invented a
machine which would take six serial x-ray photographs at the rate
of one a second, and we are lucky in having with us Professor
J. Leigh Collis, who used this apparatus and in fact injected the
opaque material into many patients. You can see this apparatus
and prints of films taken on it.

We are pleased to see our visitors from abroad, particularly
Dr. F. Henry Ellis from Boston, here for the third time. He will
keep you in order, and I now ask him to take the chair and conduct
the morning's meeting.

CONTENTS

PART V
Circulatory Support using the Intra-aortic balloon
(Chairman: Mr D Watson, Leeds)

Part I

CONSERVATION OF THE MITRAL VALVE

LONG-TERM FOLLOW-UP AFTER BJORK-SHILEY PROSTHETIC MITRAL VALVE REPLACEMENT

VIKING O. BJORK

PROFESSOR OF THORACIC AND CARDIOVASCULAR SURGERY

KAROLINSKA HOSPITAL, STOCKHOLM, SWEDEN

Two types of artificial valve are available for mitral valve replacement; high profile ball valves or low profile disc valves. The low profile disc valves are preferred because the cage of a ball valve may impinge on the ventricular septum and cause arrythmia and the ball may cause left ventricular outflow obstruction and in cases of aortic insufficiency, a mitral stenosis may be produced.

The two types of occluder are the overlapping, where the occluder hits a seat at closure every heart beat (Starr-Edwards, Lillehei-Kaster) and the non-overlapping, where the occluder fits within the ring and does not hit the seat at each heart beat, (Smeloff-Cutter, Bjork-Shiley). The latter produces less trauma to the red blood corpuscles. (Fig.1)

These two principles have been compared in a special test machine constructed by Henze, where a small amount of human blood passes back and forth through the valve due to the movement of rubber membranes. Therefore the only trauma to red blood corpuscles is due to the valve prosthesis. Both the overlapping ball and disc valves showed twice as much red cell destruction as the non-overlapping Smeloff-Cutter and Bjork-Shiley.

The increase in red cell production necessary to prevent anaemia after valve replacement was calculated for single, double, and triple valve replacement and was for the Bjork-Shiley valve only one third of that for the Starr-Edwards, and half of that for the Lillehei-Kaster. If two or three valves are replaced, it becomes important to use the valve which has the least amount of

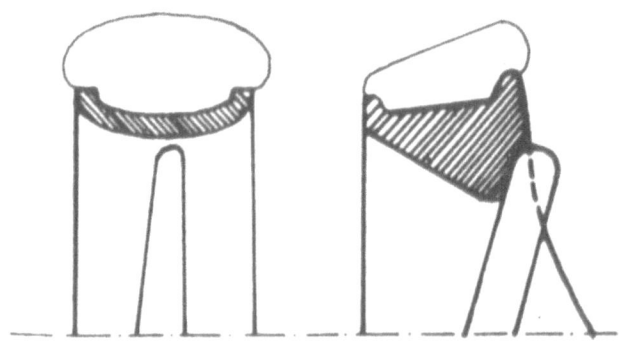

Figure 1

Diagram of an Overlapping (above) and Non-Overlapping (below) disc

blood trauma, as critical haemolysis, leading to haemolytic anaemia, may occur after multiple valve replacement with the overlapping type.

The Bjork-Shiley tilting disc valve has now been used 1023 times at the Karolinska Hospital in Stockholm - 615 in the aortic, 353 in the mitral and 55 in the tricuspid area. The disc tilts open 60° and the occluder fits within the ring and gives a central nearly laminar flow. The gradient across it does not diminish if it is opened more, even at flows as high as 26 litres per minute. Wear testing of the disc of Pyrolite as well as the struts of Stellite has shown durability of many hundred years. (Fig. 2).

I have not had one single valve failure in 1023 cases over a $6\frac{1}{2}$ year period. There has been a report (personal communication) of three instances of breakage of the larger leg or strut after eight weeks, 11 weeks and 21 months - two in No. 29 and one in No. 31. This is out of 90,000 shipped valves, and of these 16,000 are No. 29 and 31.

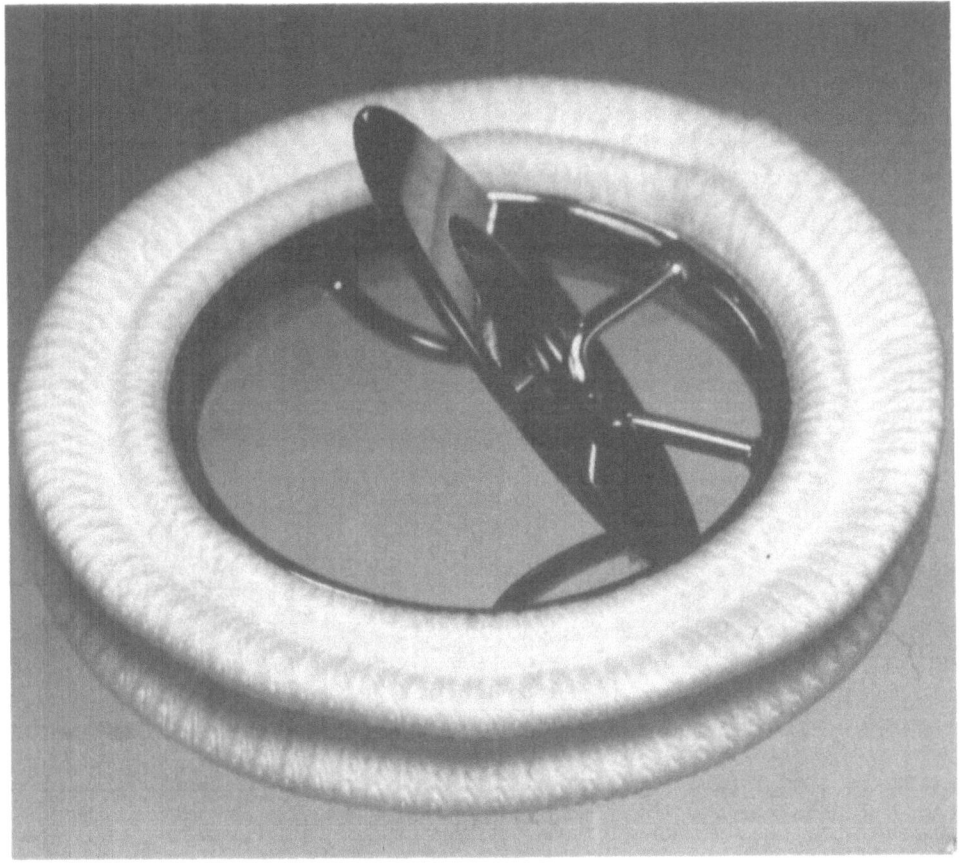

Figure 2

The Bjork-Shiley mitral valve prosthesis with a pyrolytic carbon
occluder and a double flange Teflon sewing ring.

        If at x-ray a fracture is shown on a strut, the valve has to
be exchanged as otherwise the disc will shortly embolize. A
detailed analysis of the three valves has indicated a rare
combination of factors pointing to the weld area as the probable
site of fracture. Corrective action has been taken to give even
greater safety margins, and to reduce the probability of these
fractures. The struts of 29 and 31 valves are being strengthened.
I recall that in one case during operation early in this series

I rotated the valve to give free movement of the disc, thereby
disturbing slightly the strut of the valve. The disc came loose
so I had to exchange the valve. Such a case was published,
exactly the same having happened, by Messmer and Senning. I
therefore recommend that before insertion, the valve should be
put in the valve holder and rotated ten times. This makes it
much easier to rotate, should it need rotating, once it is in
position. I also advise that you never use clamps or forceps
for this.

There is deliberate valve insufficiency due to the little
space between the disc and the ring. Its degree depends on the
difference in pressure between the left ventricle and left atrium
and the largest we can measure is around 5% of the forward stroke
volume in the largest valve.

I prefer to suture these valves as you know, by isolated
mattress sutures in the sub-annular position. Just about 20
interrupted mattress sutures. If the mitral valve has two
flanges, the sutures can be buttressed on both sides by these
suture ring flanges to prevent the sutures cutting through if
the valve base is thin, oedematous or calcified. I do recommend
placing the big hole posteriorly as it gives the smallest gradient
during higher flow, as compared to an orientation of the big
hole against the septum. The difference is not obvious at low
flows, but becomes significant at higher flows. My explanation
of this is the inward movement of the upper portion of the
ventricular septum during diastole. This narrowing of the inflow
to the left ventricle can be avoided by placing the big hole
posteriorly. Flow visualisation of this valve in Dr. Wright's
test machine in Liverpool has shown laminated flow with vortex
formation that helps to close the valve at the end of diastole.
(Figs. 3A &B, 4A &B, 5).

Eighty-three cases of isolated mitral valve replacement
followed 12 to 48 months, have had an early mortality of 2% and
a late mortality of 16%. The main cause of the deaths was
myocardial insufficiency in 10% and thrombo-embolism in 6%.
The total thrombo-embolism was 4 cases during 1,000 patient months.
Of those 6% were fatal and 4% non-fatal, 1% occurred during operation,
1% had recurrent embolism with 4 episodes and 5% had thrombotic
encapsulation of the disc. One of the four patients was
successfully operated on with simple thrombectomy from the valve
with a nerve hook and strong suction during stepwise rotation of
the valve, utilising the valve holder.

The actuarial curve shows an 89% 4-year survival with most
deaths occurring within the first year, and freedom from thrombo-
embolism of 94% after 4 years. All patients are anti-coagulated.

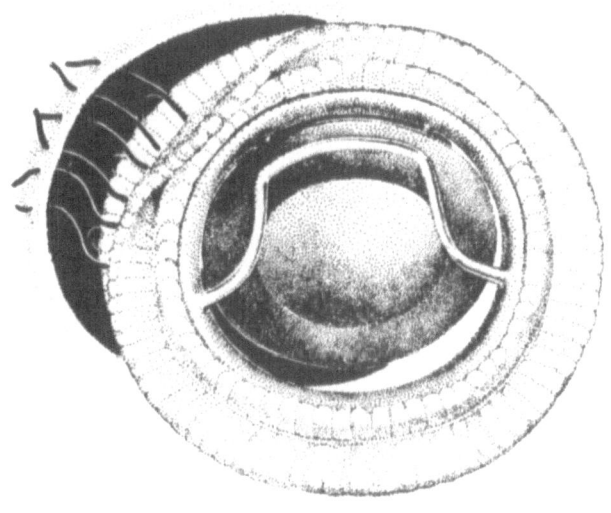

Figure 3A

The mattress sutures are passed first through the sewing ring and
then through the rim of the mitral valve from the ventricular side,
starting in the anterolateral commissure, going first anteriorly.
The big hole is oriented against the posterior wall of the left
ventricle.

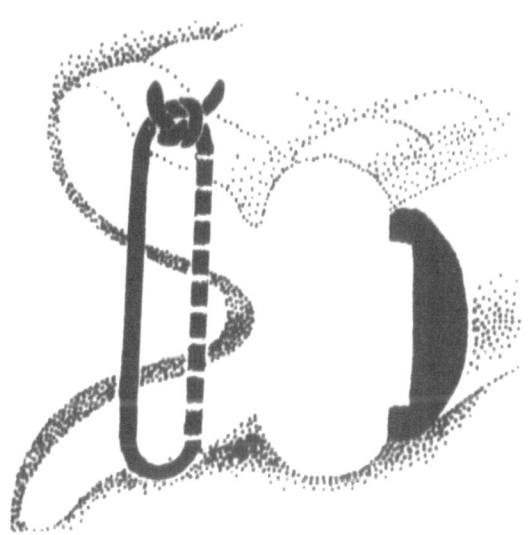

Figure 3B

The two flanges used to buffer the sutures on both sides of the
valve base.

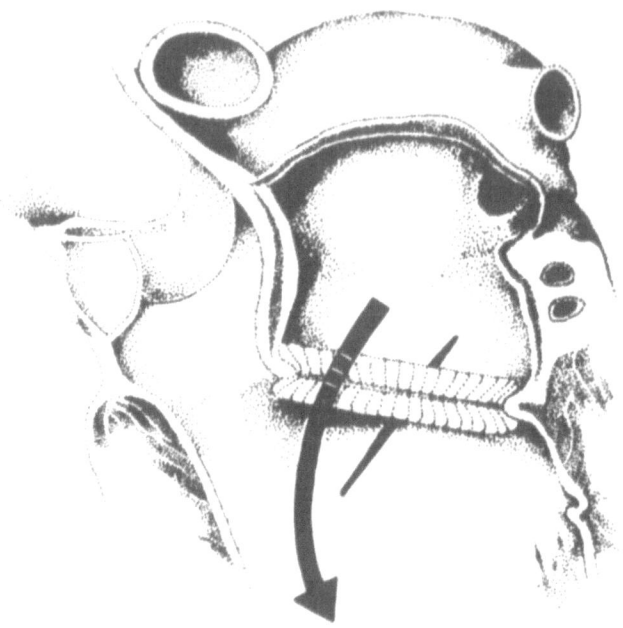

Figure 4A

Prothesis oriented with the large opening
against the ventricular septum (group I).

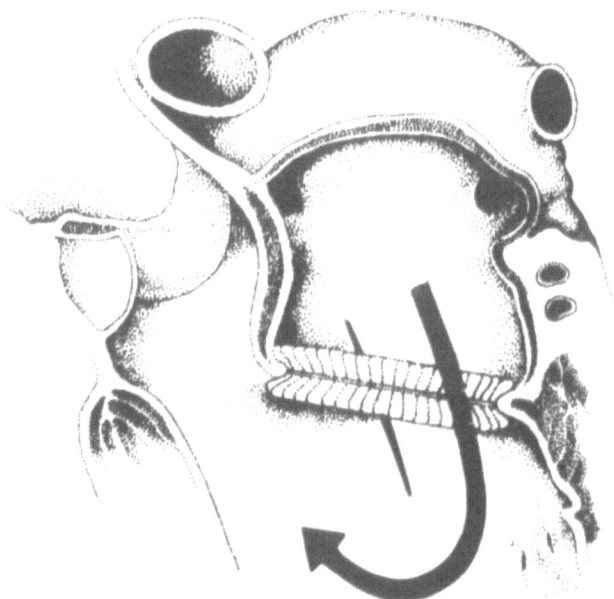

Figure 4B

Prothesis with the preferred orientation with the large opening
against the posterior wall of the left ventricle (group II).

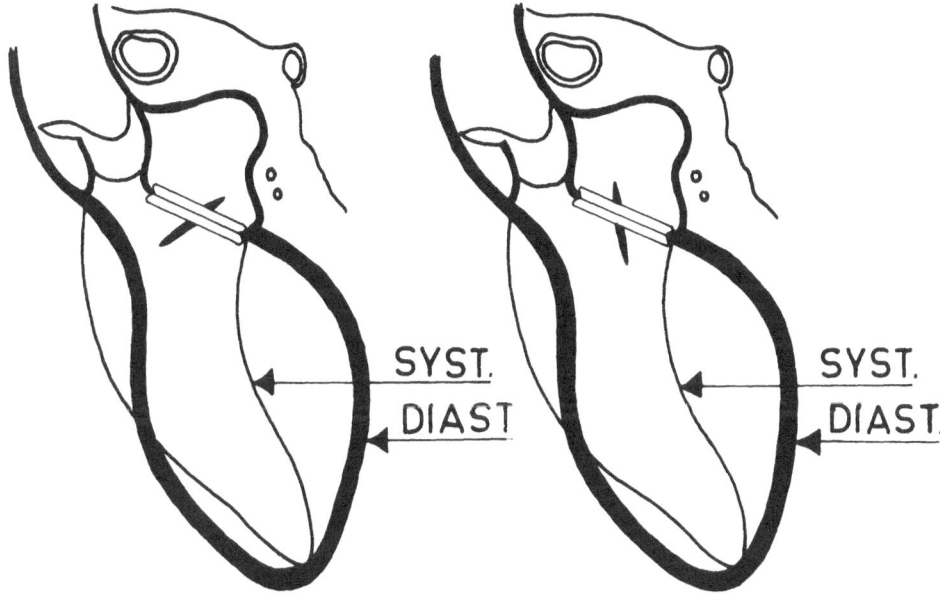

Figure 5

Diagram of the movements of the ventricular septum during the
cardiac cycle. With the anterior orientation of the big hole
(to the left), the inflow of blood into the left ventricle is
somewhat narrowed. With the posterior orientation of the big
hole (to the right), the bulging ventricular septum will not
narrow the inflow to the left ventricle.

Of the surviving patients 96% showed a subjective improvement,
which could only be proved by function tests in 80%.

    Sixty-five patients with the Bjork-Shiley valve in the mitral
position had a careful investigation at rest and during exercise,
with simultaneous recordings of the left atrial pressure and the
left ventricular pressure for calculation of the mean diastolic
pressure difference across the mitral valve. The stroke volume
at rest was before operation 49ml and increased after operation
to 53ml. During exercise the stroke volume increased from 47ml
preoperatively to 72ml postoperatively, which means a significant
increase of the stroke volume, especially pronounced during an
exercise test.

    The cardiac output showed a significant increase both at rest
and during exercise after mitral valve replacement, as assessed by
the arterio-venous oxygen difference.

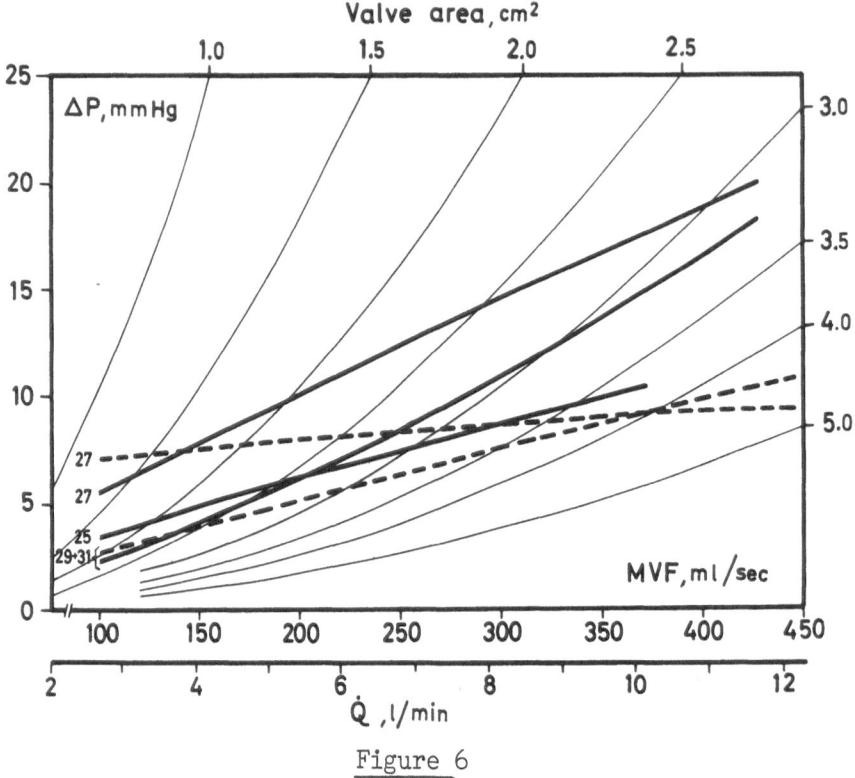

Figure 6

Driving ΔP (mm Hg), across mitral prosthesis in vivo in relation to
mitral valve flow, MVF (ml/sec), and cardiac output, Q̇ (l/min), after
mitral valve replacement at rest and during exercise. The relationship between MVF and Q̇ was obtained with least squares linear regression. Thin curved lines indicate valve area lines (cm^2) using the
Gorlin formula, which assumes a squared relationship between ΔP and
MVF. ━━: least squares regression for the observations in group I
with orientation of the large hole anterior against the ventricular
septum (26 patients) for the different prosthesis sizes; ‑‑‑: least
squares regression for the observations in group II with orientation
of the large hole posterior against the posterior wall of the left
ventricle (24 patients). The 29 mm and the 31 mm prostheses have the
same orifice area.

The relationship between the driving pressure and the flow for
the different sizes of prosthesis is shown in Fig.6. The mitral
valve flow is given both in ml/sec as well as compared to the
cardiac output in l/min. The gradient at rest is below 5mm/Hg
and during an exercise test below 10mm/Hg. The left ventricular
end diastolic pressure was at the upper limit of what can be
considered normal at rest and normal during exercise, both before
and after surgery. The left atrial pressure showed a significant
decrease at rest and a highly significant decrease after operation
during an exercise test.

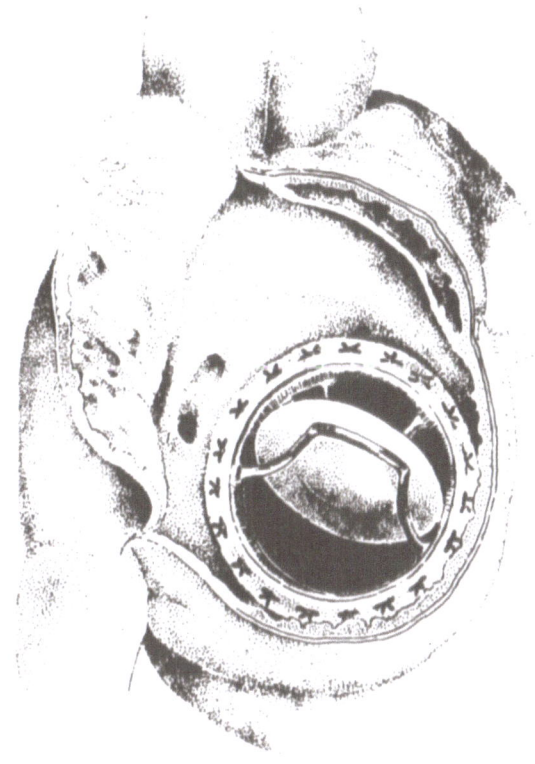

Figure 7

In the tricuspid area the large opening should be oriented against
the diaphragmatic surface of the right ventricle.

The factors determining the elevation of the left atrial
pressure after mitral valve replacement were the properties of
the valve prosthesis. The v-wave in the left atrium was
markedly elevated before operation both at rest and during
exercise and there was a significant decrease post-operatively.
However, there still remains a rather pronounced v-wave after
operation - at rest 23mm Hg and during exercise 37 mmHg. The
factor causing this v-wave must be myocardial as mitral valve
incompetence was excluded by left ventricular angiocardiography
both at rest and during an exercise test and we have seen a high
v-wave after aortic valve replacement in cases with a normal
mitral valve and a stiff myocardium. The systolic pressure in
the right ventricle was significantly decreased both at rest
and during exercise and diminished the after-load on the right
ventricle after valve replacement. The right atrial pressure,

however, did not change after mitral valve replacement. The
pulmonary vascular resistance was markedly reduced at rest and
during exercise by these mitral valve replacements. This
decrease was accompanied with a rise of cardiac output since
both aortic and right atrial pressures remained essentially
unchanged.

The Bjork-Shiley valve in the tricuspid area should be
oriented with the large opening to the diaphragmatic surface
of the right ventricle. (Fig. 7).

REFERENCES

Bjork, V.O., 1969. A new tilting disc valve prosthesis. Scand.
J.Thor.Cardiovasc.Surg 3:1.
Bjork, V.O., 1970. The central flow tilting disc valve prosthesis
(Bjork-Shiley) for mitral valve replacement. Scand.J.Thor.
Cardiovasc.Surg. 4:15.
Bjork, V.O., 1972. The pyrolytic carbon occluder for the Bjork-
Shiley tilting disc valve prosthesis. Scand.J.Thor.Cardiovasc.
Surg. 6:109.
Bjork, V.O., Book, K., Cernigliaro, C., and Holmgren, A. 1973.
The Bjork-Shiley tilting disc valve in isolated mitral lesions.
Scand. J.Thor.Carciovasc. Surg. 7:131.
Bjork, V.O., Book, K., and Holmgren, A., 1973. Significance of
position and opening angle of the Bjork-Shiley tilting disc in
mitral surgery. Scand.J.Thor.Cardiovasc.Surg. 7:187.
Book, K., Holmgren, A., and Szamosi, A., 1973. The left atrial
v-wave after mitral valve replacement. Scand.J.Thor.Cardiovasc.
Surg. 9:9.
Book, K., 1974. Mitral valve replacement with the Bjork-Shiley
tilting disc valve. Scand.J.Thor.Cardiovasc.Surg.Suppl.12.
Messmer, B.J., Okies, J.E., Hallman, G.L., and Cooley, D.A.,
1971. Mitral valve replacement with the Bjork-Shiley tilting
disc prosthesis. J.Thor.Cardiov.Surg. 62:938.
Messmer, B.J., Okies, J.E., Hallman, G.L., and Cooley, D.A.,
1972. Early and late thrombo-embolic complication after mitral
valve replacement. J.Cardiovasc.Surg. 13:281.

RUPTURED CHORDAE TENDINEAE OF THE MITRAL VALVE

M. V. BRAIMBRIDGE, B. A. ROSS, M. DAVIES

DEPARTMENT OF CARDIOTHORACIC SURGERY

ST. THOMAS'S HOSPITAL & DEPARTMENT OF PATHOLOGY
ST. GEORGE'S HOSPITAL, LONDON

The clinical problems associated with ruptured chordae tendineae of the mitral valve present in three ways: rupture of chordae to a posterior (mural) leaflet of the mitral valve which is otherwise of normal size, rupture of chordae to the anterior (aortic) leaflet, and chordal rupture associated with the redundant cusp (floppy valve) syndrome. Rupture of papillary muscles in myocardial infarction is not considered in this presentation.

1. RUPTURED POSTERIOR CHORDAE TENDINEAE IN AN OTHERWISE NORMAL VALVE

When the mitral valve is of normal size and the central chordae of the posterior leaflet rupture, the cusp rises as a hood and directs the jet of regurgitant blood anteriorly against the atrial septum and towards the base of the heart. (Fig.1).

Ten patients have been operated on at St. Thomas's Hospital between 1966 and 1971. One, the first, died of cerebral air embolism with a competent mitral valve. The nine remaining patients form the subject of this report.

Their ages were between 45 and 66 (mean 56) with six men and three women. All patients were dyspnoeic on exertion, all but one being grade III (NYHA).

Six patients were in sinus rhythm before surgery and all demonstrated the typical harsh pansystolic murmur radiating medially towards the base of the heart. A third sound was recorded in all patients.

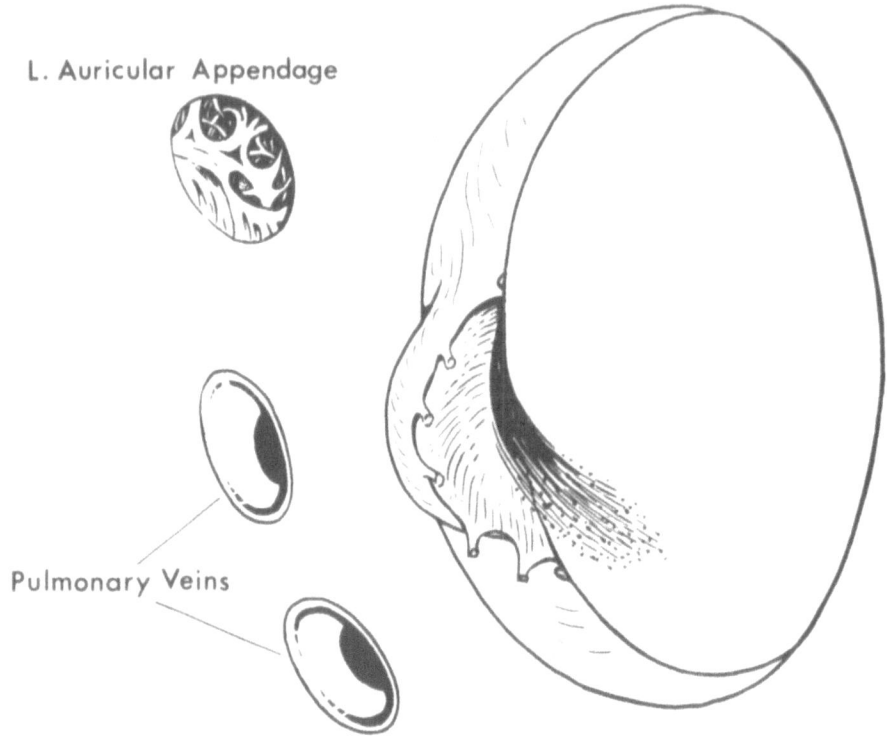

L. Auricular Appendage

Pulmonary Veins

Figure 1
The hood of the posterior cusp with ruptured chordae. The jet is
directed against the atrial septum.

        The chest radiograph showed some cardiac enlargement in seven
patients, but was never gross with a small or only slightly
enlarged left atrium. The lung fields showed prominent upper lobe
veins, but no intracardiac calcification.

        Cardiac catheterisation was carried out in all patients, but
one collapsed during investigation and the procedure was abandoned.
Three of the remaining eight patients showed a systolic wave in
the left atrial or pulmonary wedge tracing of 60mm/Hg or more, while
the remainder had systolic waves around 30mm/Hg. In six cases left
ventricular angiography was performed to confirm the severity of
the mitral regurgitation.

a.   Operation Technique

        At operation through a median sternotomy a systolic thrill was
felt impinging on the interatrial septum. Bypass was instituted

and the left atrium opened behind the interatrial groove. The characteristic hood formed by elongation of the unsupported part of the cusp was seen at operation.

The McGoon operation as modified by Gerbode [2,3] was used to correct the defect in each case. The edges of the cusp still attached to chordae were approximated using interrupted Lembert sutures as horizontal mattress sutures. (Fig.2). The flail part of the leaflet was inverted onto the ventricular surface and the sutures were continued for 3-4cms., onto the left atrial wall, plicating the valve ring at this point. These sutures were supported by interrupted 4/0 sutures.

After careful venting of the heart to prevent air embolism and discontinuing of bypass, the dominant systolic wave in the left atrial pressure trace disappeared and the mean left atrial pressure fell towards normal. In addition the systolic thrill could no longer be felt.

All patients were anticoagulated for six weeks to reduce the risk of venous thrombosis and pulmonary embolism.

b. Follow-Up

All nine patients have been seen and critically reviewed one to six years (mean 3.3 years) after operation. Six of the patients have been seen by an independent cardiologist. The remaining three declined to attend the hospital and asked to be assessed by their local cardiologist.

Exertional dyspnoea has been graded I-IV in all but one, and after operation eight patients led a normal life with minimal disability. One patient had a grade II effort intolerance but he also suffered from obstructive airways disease. This patient had no detectable murmur and he performed well on the bicycle ergometer.

Six patients were in sinus rhythm before operation. These remained so and a further patient who was previously in atrial fibrillation reverted to sinus rhythm after operation. A third sound was noted in all patients prior to surgery but this subsequently disappeared in each case.

The apical pansystolic murmurs were graded from 1-4. Before operation all had grade 3 or 4 murmurs. After operation two patients had normal heart sounds with no murmur and six had only a soft grade 1/4 murmur. One patient's murmur was graded 2/4 but he performed excellently on the bicycle and his effort intolerance was only grade I.

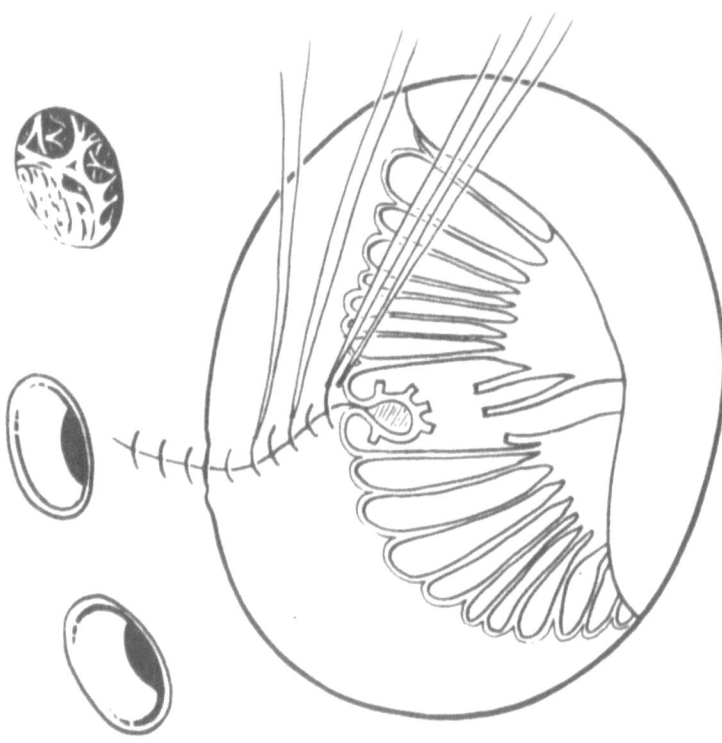

Figure 2
The plicated segment of posterior cusp with the plication running
across the valve annulus into the atrium.

        The six patients seen at St. Thomas's were assessed on the
bicycle ergometer and were asked to perform as much work as they
were reasonably able. All except one maintained quite strenuous
exercise of at least two minutes at 600 kpm/min, and the resulting
dyspnoea was only moderate. The single poor response was seen in
the youngest of the group. She was not disabled symptomatically
(grade I) and had only a grade 1/4 murmur, but could only manage
one minute at 600 kpm/min. This poor degree of exercise may be
related to her low body weight.

        There was a significant reduction in heart size comparing
chest x-rays before and after operation. All postoperative films
showed a heart size within normal limits and there was a
significant reduction in the size of those hearts that were
previously enlarged.

        The cardiologist did not consider it ethically justifiable to

recatheterise any one of such fit patients and thus there are no
haemodynamic data to report. Patients still in atrial fibrillation
continue with Digoxin and two patients still take small doses of
diuretics.

Thus 89 per cent of these patients lead virtually normal lives
as a result of the valve repair and there has been no deterioration
in any case during the period of follow up.

2.   RUPTURE OF CHORDAE TENDINEAE TO THE ANTERIOR LEAFLET

Rupture of chordae tendineae to the anterior leaflet has been
found by almost all surgeons to be uncorrectable by a plastic
procedure and valve replacement has proved essential. At
St. Thomas's Hospital five patients have been operated on for
anterior chordal rupture and all have been treated by Starr-Edwards
prosthetic valve replacement. All patients are still alive with
minimal dyspnoea, but one has since developed a cerebral embolus.

3.   RUPTURED CHORDAE ASSOCIATED WITH THE REDUNDANT CUSP

Ruptured chordae, when they are part of the "redundant cusp"
"floppy valve" "midsystolic click late systolic murmur syndrome"
form a different surgical problem.

a.   Pathological Features

The characteristic pathological feature of the redundant cusp
syndrome is expansion and thickening of the valve leaflets. They
become ballooned and floppy with the chordae tendineae attenuated
and weakened when they may rupture. At a late stage a fibrous
swelling may develop on the adjacent endocardial surface and this
can aggregate with the chordae to form a fusion lesion.

Microscopically this is a degenerative disease. The primary
process is a fibrous disintegration which begins at the tip of
the fibrous core of the leaflet and extends outwards towards the
annulus and into the chordae tendineae (Fig.3). Floppy valves
were found in 5 per cent of 249 routine post mortem studies carried
out by one of us (M.D.) at St. George's Hospital. The incidence
increases with age. There were no cases below the age of 40. In
the fifth decade the incidence was 2.5 per cent: in the sixth and
seventh decade, 4.7 per cent: in the eighth 6 per cent and in
patients over 80, 8 per cent.

The pathological redundant cusp syndrome is synonymous in the
literature with the clinical mid-systolic click and late systolic
murmur syndrome. The natural history is usually benign with mitral
regurgitation occurring only at a late stage. Leatham (1973)

studied 62 patients with moderate late systolic murmurs. 50 per cent of these had a mid-systolic click also. Only 7 per cent showed marked deterioration during the 9-22 years of the study.

From the large number of patients who have the redundant cusp syndrome, any surgical series is necessarily involved with only those few who deteriorate. The reasons for early deterioration are ruptured chordae - the most common - sub-acute bacterial endocarditis and the association with a generalised connective disease such as cystic medial degeneration, Marfan's syndrome, Ehlers Danlos syndrome and osteogenesis imperfecta, which produce weakening and dilatation of the valve annulus. The pathological features of these conditions are separate from those of the redundant cusp syndrome where the primary process is in the valve leaflet. The increased strain produced by the heavy floppy cusps summates with the effects of the weakened annulus to produce dilatation and early regurgitation.

b.   Surgical Series at St. Thomas's Hospital

Sixteen patients with the redundant cusp syndrome underwent operation at St. Thomas's Hospital between 1965 and 1972. Twelve were male and four female aged 49-67 with an average age of 58.3 years. Fourteen patients were treated with mitral valve replacement which represented 8 per cent of the 175 mitral valve replacements performed during the same period. Two patients were treated by valvoplasty.

Eleven of the sixteen patients had ruptured chordae. Ten had ruptured posterior chordae and they presented with the sudden onset of mitral regurgitation and swift deterioration. Only one patient had anterior chordal rupture and this was limited to a few medial adherent chordae. Anterior chordal rupture occurs more frequently than this series would suggest but is usually seen in Coroners' post-mortems because it is associated with sudden death. This suggests that anterior chordal rupture is more catastrophic to mitral valve function than rupture of posterior chordae, as one would expect from the size of the cusp.

One patient had subacute bacterial endocarditis. The posterior chordae were all ruptured and vegetations were evident.

None had cystic medial degeneration but two had osteogenesis imperfecta. This disease is basically a collagen disorder which may occur with Marfan's syndrome and has similar cardiovascular complications.

c.   Clinical Features

The clinical presentation of these patients was on the whole

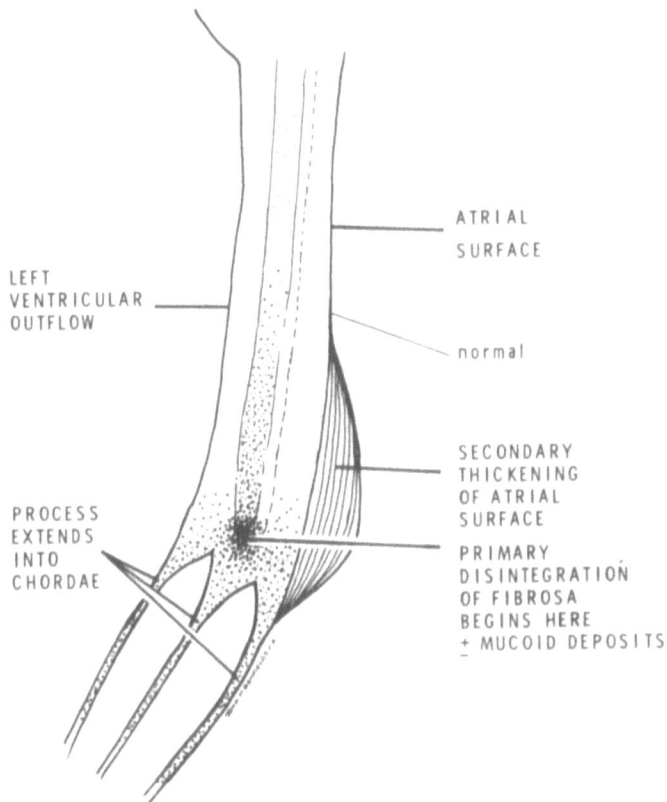

ATRIAL
SURFACE

LEFT
VENTRICULAR
OUTFLOW

normal

PROCESS
EXTENDS
INTO
CHORDAE

SECONDARY
THICKENING
OF ATRIAL
SURFACE

PRIMARY
DISINTEGRATION
OF FIBROSA
BEGINS HERE
+ MUCOID DEPOSITS
-

Figure 3
Disintegration of the fibrous core of the leaflet spreading into
the chordae.

classical. A past history of a heart murmur is commonly described
in the redundant cusp syndrome. Twelve (75%) of this series had
had such a murmur for between 8 and 50 years with an average of
26 years. In accordance with the natural history, two modes of
presentation were found. Ten patients (62%), those with posterior
chordal rupture, presented with the sudden onset of symptoms and
rapid deterioration and demanded early surgery, the earliest at
two months. The other six had a gradual onset and insiduous
progress, the longest being eight years. These patients,
therefore, could not be distinguished from other forms of mitral
regurgitation. The average duration of symptoms for the whole
group was two years. The important symptom was breathlessness.
All but one had dyspnoea grade III (NYHA) or more.

The usual clinical signs described in the redundant cusp syndrome are sinus rhythm and a mid-systolic click and late systolic murmur. In this series, however, 56 per cent were in atrial fibrillation. These were equally distributed between the long and short history patients. Only one patient had a mid-systolic click and late systolic murmur. All the remainder when presented for surgery had pansystolic murmurs and therefore could not be distinguished from other forms of mitral regurgitation. 13 patients (81%) had a third sound.

Echocardiography, so useful in the diagnosis of this syndrome, was not employed in any case as the latest patient in this series was operated on in 1972. The chest x-rays of this group were compared with those of all others undergoing mitral valve replacement during the same period. The mean cardiothoracic ratio was 58% in the redundant cusp series compared with 66% in the others. Left atrial enlargement was also rather less - 94% had grade 1-2/4 enlargement compared with 71% of the other mitral valve replacements and only 6% were markedly enlarged compared with 29%. Cardiac catheterisation was performed in all patients but no distinguishing features were found.

d. Operative Technique

14 patients had Starr valve replacements while two had valvoplasties. One valvoplasty was carried out ill advisedly on the first patient in this series due to our inexperience with this condition. The second was on a patient with osteogenesis imperfecta in whom a blood coagulation defect was present and anticoagulants were contraindicated.

Several operative techniques have been described to prevent the high reported incidence of prosthetic valve dehiscence in this condition. Cooley reports a hospital mortality of 8 per cent because of dehiscence [8] and Austen reports an incidence of 8 per cent in his follow up cases [9]. In this series carefully spaced interrupted sutures of 2/0 Tevdek were passed through the flimsy valve annulus and then as a vertical mattress through the prosthetic valve ring (Fig. 4). This provided a maximal depth of contact between the annulus and the sewing ring. Many more sutures were used than in other mitral valve replacements, an average of 42 compared with 31.

e. Results

There were no operative deaths. One patient died $3\frac{1}{2}$ years after surgery from trachial obstruction following an epistasis while asleep. His prothrombin time, incidentally, was well controlled at that time. Morbidity included six patients who

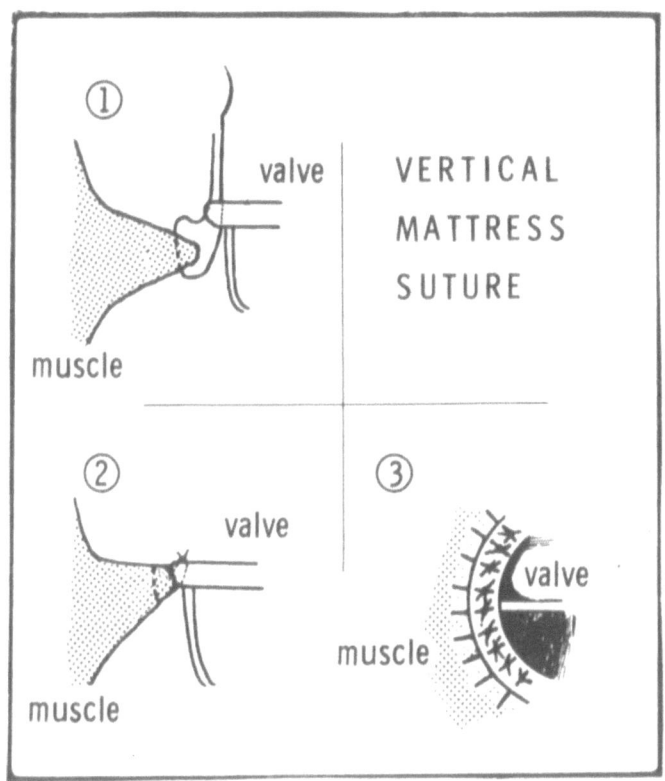

Figure 4

Multiple vertical mattress sutures used in this area

developed persistent ventricular ectopics and were treated with procaineamide. Two tracheostomies were performed on patients early in the series in the two cases of osteogenesis imperfecta who had the anticipated bleeding problems postoperatively.

The 15 survivors have been followed up for from six months to six years with an average of two years. 13 have no or trivial exercise intolerance: two have definite effort intolerance, these were the two patients who had ill advised McGoon valvoplasties. Two patients have pansystolic murmurs - also the two patients with valvoplasties.

4. CONCLUSIONS

The experience derived from these series of patients with ruptured chordae operated on at St. Thomas's Hospital suggest that all such patients can be safely and satisfactorily treated surgically. Those with ruptured chordae of the posterior cusp associated with normal sized cusps can be well managed with the modified McGoon cusp and ring plication operation. Those with rupture of the chordae to the anterior cusp and those with posterior ruptured chordae associated with the redundant cusp, floppy valve syndrome are best treated in our hands by mitral valve replacement. The operative mortality of all these groups can be expected to be low and follow up satisfactory.

REFERENCES

1. Brown, A.H., Braimbridge, M.V., Clement, A.J., Sabar, E., and Mendel, D (1968). Valvoplasty for abnormalities of the posterior (mural) cusp of the mitral valve. Thorax 23,608.

2. Gerbode, F., Kerth, W.J., Kelly, J.J., and Selzer, A. (1966). The surgical correction of mitral insufficiency due to ruptured chordae tendineae. Bul.Soc.int.Chir., 25.483.

3. McGoon, D.C., (1960). Repair of mitral insufficiency due to ruptured chordae tendineae. J.Thorac.Cardiovasc.Surg. 39,357.

4. Frable, W.J., (1969). Mucinous degeneration of the cardiac valves: The "Floppy Valve" Syndrome. J.Thorac.Cardiovasc. Surg. 58,62.

5. Davis, R.H., Schuster, B., Knoebel, S.B., and Fisch, D. (1971). Myxomatous degeneration of the mitral valve. Amer. J.Cardiol. 28,449.

6. Hill, D.G., Davies, M.J., and Braimbridge, M.V., (1974). The natural history and surgical management of the redundant cusp syndrome (floppy mitral valve). J.Thoracic.Cardiovasc. Surg. 67,519.

7. Wood, S.J., Thomas, J., and Braimbridge, M.V. (1973). Mitral valve disease and open heart surgery in osteogenesis imperfecta tarda. Brit.Heart J. 35,103.

8. Cooley, D.A., Gerami, S., Hallman, G.L., Wukasch, D.C., and
    Hall, R.J. (1972). Mitral insufficiency due to myxomatous
    transformation:"floppy valve" syndrome. J.Cardiovasc.Surg.
    13,346.

9. Sanders, C.A., Austen, W.G. Harthorne, J.W., Dinsmore, R.E.,
    and Scannell, J.G. (1967). Diagnosis and Surgical treatment
    of mitral regurgitation due to ruptured chordae tendineae.
    New Engl.J.Med. 276,943.

10. Allen, H., Harris, A., Leatham, A. Natural history of
    slight mitral regurgitation. Brit.HeartJ. 1973,35,552.

THE TREATMENT OF MITRAL STENOSIS

MAGDI H. YACOUB

CONSULTANT CARDIAC SURGEON

HAREFIELD HOSPITAL, HAREFIELD, UXBRIDGE, MIDDLESEX

We believe that the best operation on the mitral valve is a conservative restorative one, and this has been our policy for the last six years. Table I shows that 695 patients underwent mitral valve operations during the period from August 1969 to August 1975. Of these, 493 underwent mitral valve replacement, and 202 had conservative operations. The conservative operations were all open operations and were for predominant stenosis in 158 and for predominant regurgitation in 44. Most of the latter belonged to the "floppy valve" syndrome group of patients and some were in the congenital age group. During the first two years of this period it was our policy to replace the mitral valve for the "floppy valve" syndrome, but during the last three years we have repaired such valves with ruptured chordae to the anterior and posterior cusps.

It has been mentioned in the past that one of the great dangers of performing open mitral valvotomy was the risk of replacing the valve. We have found the opposite to be true. Very quickly we adopted the policy of performing all mitral operations open, and we now find that we conserve more valves than we used to. Fig. 1 relates the percentage of patients undergoing open mitral valvotomy, with or without repair, to the total number of patients undergoing mitral valve surgery during each year. Six years ago approximately 25% of valves were conserved, but lately that figure has reached 36% and even 74%.

The technique we use is fairly simple. The valve is exposed on cardio pulmonary bypass and clots and fibrinous deposits are removed from the commissures. The commissures are then sharply divided with a knife to the ring at the two fibrous trigones. No

TABLE I

OPERATIONS ON THE MITRAL VALVE

(Harefield Hospital, August 1969-August 1975)

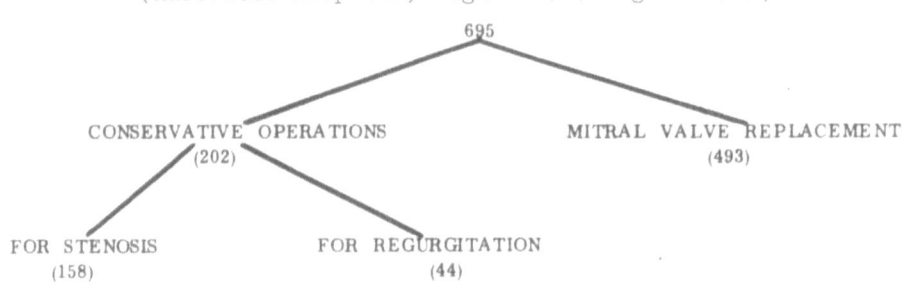

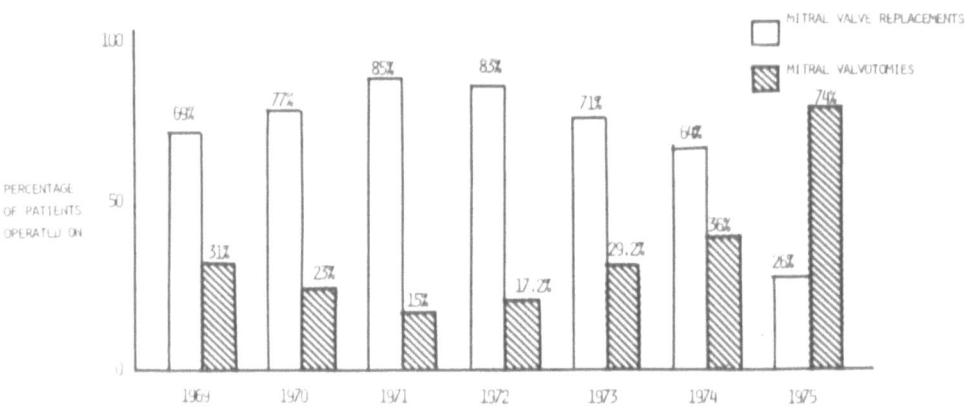

Figure 1.   Percentage number of mitral valve replacements compared
            to mitral valvotomy operations.

attempt is made at stretching the valve before dividing the commissures. Next a Tubbs' dilator is used to separate the sub-valvar mechanism and the valve is inspected again. If there is still sub-valvar fusion, as is commonly the case, the papillary muscles are divided way into the ventricle. Lastly the mobility of the valve is tested. We do not regard fusion of the papillary muscle directly onto the cusp as a contraindication to a conservative operation. Splitting the valve with a dilator commonly produces a tear in the posterior cusp and this is why the cusps are always divided with a knife. I believe that an open operation allows one to produce the best possible relief of valvar and sub-valvar stenosis. In the past we used to consider gross thickening and shortening of the chordae to be absolute contraindications to a conservative operation but now we divide the commissures and papillary muscles and test the valve. This is done using a method very similar to the one previously described by Mr. Yates. We believe that it is important not to subject the left ventricle to any pressure until it is beating actively, so we clamp the aorta, put a cannula into the aortic root and wait until the heart is beating actively. Sometimes we inject some calcium chloride at this point. Only when the heart is beating actively is it subjected to pressure from another cannula at the apex. We have found this a much better way of detecting leaks than by injecting saline through the valve. It is also possible by this technique to establish exactly where the leak is. If it is central one will want to elevate the posterior cusp. If it is due to an unstable part of the valve mechanism then that part will have to be fixed or overlapped by some sort of annuloplasty.

Of the 158 patients who underwent open mitral valvotomy, with or without annuloplasty, most were in the fourth to sixth decades, but one was a four months old child with a parachute valve. A conservative procedure was found to be possible. All these patients were symptomatic with clear clinical evidence of severe mitral stenosis. The preoperative catheter findings are summarised in Table II.

Approximately 10% of the patients had had a previous closed valvotomy but this did not constitute a contraindication to another attempt at valvotomy. Calcification detected before operation by x-ray or echocardiogram did not constitute a contraindication either. Extensive calcification was found in 15% of the cases and this was removed at operation. Sometimes large amounts of calcium had to be removed from the commissures before the mobility of the valve could be properly assessed. Atrial clot was found in seven patients and fibrinous deposits found on the valve in six. These fibrinous deposits are not uncommon and I am surprised they do not give rise to more emboli

TABLE II

PRE-OPERATIVE CATHETER FINDINGS

PARAMETER	MEAN	RANGE
Mean Pulmonary Wedge	18mm/Hg	3-32mm/Hg
Mean Pulmonary Artery	27mm/Hg	6-80mm/Hg
Cardiac Index	2.3 Litres	1.4-3.7 Litres
Pulmonary Vascular Resistance	2.6 Units	0.5-15 Units

TABLE III

OTHER PROCEDURES AT TIME OF MITRAL VALVOTOMY

158 PATIENTS

PROCEDURE	NO.	%
Mitral Annuloplasty	56	35.4%
Homograft Replacement of Aortic Valve	23	14.6%
Decortication of Left Atrium	6	3.8%
Coronary Artery Bypass Graft	4	2.5%
Tricuspid Valvotomy	4	2.5%
Atrial Septal Defect	1	0.6%
TOTAL:	94	59.5%

Table IV

EARLY   AND   LATE   MORTALITY   FOLLOWING   MITRAL   VALVOTOMY

158 Patients   Follow Up   3-72 Months

OPERATION	NO. OF PATIENTS	EARLY		LATE		TOTAL	
		NO.	%	NO.	%	NO.	%
Isolated Valvotomy	64	0	0%	1	1.6%	1	1.6%
Valvotomy and AVR (Homograft)	23	0	0%	2	8.7%	2	8.7%
Valvotomy and Decortication of LA	6	2	33%	0	0%	2	33%
Total No. of Patients	158	2	1.3%	3	1.9%	5	3.2%

during closed valvotomy. Sometimes there is massive left atrial clot and this chamber has to be decorticated. For these patients operation carries a high risk.

Table III lists the additional procedures required in this group of patients having open mitral valvotomy. Note that 56 patients out of the 158 had an additional annuloplasty. In all 60% of the patients needed something more than a valvotomy.

Table IV shows in detail the early and late operative mortality in these patients. There were two early deaths, early death being defined as any death occurring within six weeks of the operation. Both occurred in the group of six patients who had to have decortication of the left atrium and both were due to the low output state. In the isolated valvotomy group there was one late death

At the end of 72 months 96% of the 158 patients were alive and that is as good, if not better, than any series of valve replacements.

The post-operative assessment has been clinical. 91% profess to be improved, 2.1% to be the same, and 3.5% to be worse. A systolic murmur was present in 25% of them but only five patients had important mitral regurgitation.

In conclusion we believe that open valvotomy is the best form of treatment for mitral stenosis and open valvotomy with or without annuloplasty offers better results than a closed procedure.

DISCUSSION

CHAIRMAN: F. HENRY ELLIS

LAHEY CLINIC, BOSTON, MASSACHUSETTS, U.S.A.

CHAIRMAN: Combined stenosis and insufficiency problems, I
guess you would agree, are best treated by replacement, so shall
we start with mitral stenosis and get things moving. I would
like to ask Mr. Braimbridge if there is a place any longer for
closed mitral valvotomy, or should all mitral stenosis patients
be operated on using open techniques?

BRAIMBRIDGE: I think this is a very interesting problem
still, because those of us brought up in the older days learned
to use closed mitral valvotomy and this is no longer true. The
one operation I do not like to leave my senior registrar doing
alone now is a closed mitral valvotomy. We have had one case
die, and one or two problems I have had to rush in to. A lot of
the new young men feel very insecure with closed mitral valvotomy.
The one snag as I see it about open mitral valvotomy is that when
it comes to having to do the valve replacement one has, to a
certain extent, queered the operative pitch. I changed to open
mitral valvotomy for two years, thinking that I was old-fashioned
doing closed mitral valvotomy, and then analysed the series at the
end of it. I found that I had a slightly higher incidence of
pansystolic murmur following open mitral valvotomy than after
closed. I also found the logistic load was greater doing an open
rather than a closed procedure in our small unit, and have gone
back in the average case to doing a closed procedure so that one
can have a very simple procedure for the second stage. I think
that what has probably changed this now is that the reparative
procedures are much better - that everyone is tenting the valves
better and are tailoring the valvotomy much better and can do
what Mr. Yacoub has described, sewing up the places that are
leaking and mobilising the chordae. An open mitral valvotomy

31

today is very different from what it was five years ago, but
basically I, and a lot of the surgeons in smaller units such
as ours, are still doing closed mitral valvotomy with good
results, and I am sure that there is still a place for it.

CHAIRMAN: Do the other members of the panel agree with
what has just been said?

BJORK: Well, I do not feel old-fashioned, but we still use
the trans-ventricular dilatation, but first after having seen
from a left ventricular angiogram that it is an ideal case, which
means moveable, thin cusps that are fused in the commissure. We
can see in suitable cases on the angiogram the long distance to
the papillary muscle. In those cases when the fashion was to do
everything open, we did several open, but used the dilator and
then saw what little more we could do with dissection and it
was extraordinary in a case with thin cusps it was not necessary
to do more once I had used the dilator. The trick was never to
open it more than 3.5cm for a woman and 4cm for a man, then
nothing wrong happened; it always ruptured in the commissure.
There were not many of those cases, but now when we see a
suitable case we use trans-ventricular dilatation, and think we
get as good a result as we can with the open. The other cases
are more complicated. I still cannot understand how if you have
a thick valve that you open that you can lessen the gradient.
We will have to find out in the long run whether conservative
treatment, with cutting through the papillary muscle that is
fixed on the rear of the valve, etc., that you can really get
enough cusp movement to get the gradient down on an exercise
test. You can certainly get the patient to survive and you can
get rid of insufficiency, but I will see if that patient four
or five years afterwards will feel as good. I think we have a
lot more calcium involved in our cases, anyway more rheumatic
fever perhaps.

CHAIRMAN: Do I interpret you correctly Professor Bjork,
that you place more reliance on the ventriculogram than you do
on the clinical findings as far as the pliability of the valve
is concerned?

BJORK: Well, always before advising a closed operation,
it is a must to have a ventriculogram first of all to see
mobility, and then of course, insufficiency.

CHAIRMAN: Mr. Yacoub, I gather that your concepts differ
from those of the previous speakers in that you do all of your
reconstructive operations open for mitral stenosis. Can you
tell us a word about how you are able to increase this
percentage of reconstruction as opposed to replacement, because
there is quite a striking difference between your practice and
what is happening in the States where fewer and fewer operations
are done to conserve the mitral valve.

YACOUB: I think by doing all the operations open one finds
that one learns much more about the functional anatomy of mitral

stenosis and mitral regurgitation, and one can now evaluate the valve better, and get a more aggressive approach to mobilising the fused chordae, whereas before one would be very worried about splitting the papillary muscle into the ventricle. I take Professor Bjork's point whether this is going to last or not, but certainly one can split the papillary muscle and mobilise the valve and see it move, and one can then get a valve which is fully mobile and also is competent, much more so than previously, when we tended to take a valve out if it looked fused.

DYDE: May I put a completely opposing point of view? I am very unhappy about mitral valvotomy. I have operated on 62 patients with the idea of doing an open mitral valvotomy. In a third of those I have immediately excised the valve on looking at it. In another third I have done some form of dissection and then gone on to some form of annuloplasty, and then in the end not been satisfied with the result because these valves seemed to be so gnarled and fibrosed and thickened that I can't conceive they will last long. And then in another third I have left the inadequate mitral valvotomy that I have done, and those patients appear, or tell me that they are satisfied with the result of the operation, but I am certainly not satisfied with leaving that valve in place, and I think the time has come now when if you can't get a perfect result with a mitral valvotomy, either open or closed, and you cannot get the sort of result when you are absolutely certain that that patient will have four or five years of good health, then I think you ought to consider putting a prosthesis in.

CHAIRMAN: Any other comments on this point?

ROSS: I disagree sir, because there are many patients coming up now who had their closed mitral valvotomy 17 years ago, and all Mr. Dyde is looking for is four or five years from a prosthesis which I don't believe is better than your own valve. One interesting point to note is on which cases to do closed mitral valvotomy. The best cases by far are young women, in sinus rhythm with no systolic murmur, no history of embolism, with a loud first sound and a good opening snap. I think then it would be quite wrong to do anything else in the first instance than a closed mitral valvotomy using, preferably, only the finger. If an expanding dilator has to be used it should be opened gradually and progressively.

BJORK: May I just say when there is a discussion like this, when we totally disagree about one thing, if we see the same patient we will probably agree. Now I don't see mitral valves in sinus rhythm, maybe one, but very seldom. Secondly, you may remember when we decalcified the aortic valves, I have been in that area, it lasted for one or two years and the calcium came back again. So if you start to decalcify a mitral valve, for instance, as I know several surgeons do to get a mobile valve, my guess is that you will have the calcium back again in a couple of years.

CHAIRMAN: What you are saying really is that the pathologic process in mitral stenosis is a progressive process regardless of

what you do technically. Eventually the valve becomes stiff and
has to be replaced, whether it is five years, ten years or 15
years.

BJORK: No, but if you hit it at that late moment when you
have calcium in it already, taking that away will not prevent it
recalcifying very quickly. We know that no-one today will do
de-calcification of an aortic valve.

TEMPLE: I was very interested in what Mr. Ross was saying,
and I do not think that any of us would really disagree with him
except in one thing; we all talk as though this disease has not
changed. Now I have got patients who did very well with mitral
valvotomy I did more than 20 years ago, and are still well - you
do not see them now, where does Mr. Ross get his 18 year old girl
with severe symptoms?

BJORK: From Persia or Iran.

TEMPLE: I have practised closed mitral valvotomy for many
years now, but am less and less satisfied with it. I am less
satisfied because they are different patients from ones I was doing
even ten years ago, a different type of valve, rheumatic fever
produces a more fibrous valve now. I think the Bjork-Shiley valve
is a lot happier than the Starr-Edwards valve because one can put
a big orifice in. The other thing is that I have always been
worried if I am going to try and do a repair because I have never
been able to adequately test whether my repair is any good. I
think Mr. Yacoub has given the answer to this, and I think on
this basis I shall exclude closed mitral valvotomy in these cases.

GRAY: I speak as a physician rather than a surgeon. I
think one point about mitral stenosis is that nobody really
imagines that closed valvotomy very often produces a perfect
result, but I think it is important that in mitral stenosis you
do not need a perfect result to abolish the gradient and relieve
the symptoms. The difference of an orifice of between $\frac{1}{2}$cm and
2cm is quite enough to make an enormous difference to the symptoms
of the patient. Would the surgeons agree with me on that?

WATSON: I would not entirely agree. The degree of rigidity
of the cusps is most important. However great the orifice produced
by the dilator if the cusps remain thick and rigid the left atrial
pressure will not fall.

MEARNS: I just wanted to raise one or two points about the
investigation of these patients. We have heard about the
effectiveness of Mr. Ross's stethoscope in assessing these valves.
Recently echocardiography is being used and you can now measure
the mobility of the anterior cusp of the valve. I wonder if
people are using this and is the valve more mobile afterwards.
Can Mr. Yacoub show that the cusps he has mobilised at open
operation are in fact more mobile afterwards?

YACOUB: Yes, we do routine echo. We found that when you
refer to mobility many people used to think that the opening
movement, the extent of the excursion, was a direct measurement

of the length of the chordae and the mobility. That is not so, and that does not change effectively. However, if you are referring to the diastolic closure rate as a measure of extent of relief of stenosis, hence mobility, then there is a significant change in the rigid valves. To get an idea about that the valve echo is very, very useful, but it only gives you one cut somewhere in the valve and this could be very misleading. A valve which appears on the echo to be very heavily calcified indeed, with just multiple thick lines, just like a myxoma, may be very mobile on one side and the echo just happens to go across a calcified lateral commissure, which is a very small localised area of calcification.

CHAIRMAN: We have a representative of Professor Senning's clinic in Zurich. Would you like to say a word?

TURINA: We have always used a closed approach similar to that which Professor Bjork has described. One point I would like to raise is that of cost. We are not a socialist country and we are under great pressure from the authorities to reduce our spending so far as is practicable, and for this reason, and also because we are short of hospital staff, we have always favoured the closed approach and found the results to be satisfactory.

CHAIRMAN: Obviously there is a great deal of difference of opinion about closed versus open versus replacement. We have several countries represented here but we have not yet heard from the United States.

McENANY: I think that our group in Boston probably does more closed valvotomies than any other in the United States, having reported recently a large series of 800 cases. Our protocol at present is to evaluate the patients with angio beforehand and select out those with high grade incompetence. The remainder are put up for closed valvotomy. Seven per cent progress to immediate open operations for one of three reasons. Firstly, finding thrombus in the left atrium; secondly, finding calcium that was not picked up in the echo; and thirdly finding severe sub-valvar disease of chordal fusion. Only about four or five times a year do we do a valve replacement for one of these reasons. There is still controversy in the United States which is very well mirrored by the discussions here, as to whether this is a bona fide operation. I think that the point that was made is very true that it is extremely hard to turn out a cardiac surgeon in the United States who is going to be very comfortable about doing closed transventricular mitral valvotomy. I think that probably in ten years nobody is going to be trained to do it. Not that it is a bad operation, but nobody knows how to do it. We think that it is a good operation with an excellent result in an appropriately chosen patient.

HOLLINRAKE: One hears a lot of talk about excellent results, good results and bad results. Has Mr. Yacoub any objective measurements?

YACOUB: Yes, we have some data but with non-invasive

techniques if you like, like chest film, echo, but we have not
catheterised them again.

BRAIMBRIDGE: Could I just make one comment there. I
believe very strongly that the assessment of the functional result
that one sees on everybody's series has to be made by a hostile
cardiologist. I learned this when I was a senior registrar and
in the case of one particular surgeon I worked for, the patient
was seen by the surgeon and by the cardiologist on the same morning
and the comment was continually made by the cardiologist who saw
the patient second, "Why did you tell the surgeon that you were
doing very well and you just told me you were not" and he said,
"Well, he is such a nice man, I did not like to disappoint him."

CHAIRMAN: Any other comments?

DYDE: There is a matter of attitude to open mitral valvotomy.
If any of the speakers have done open mitral valvotomy and they
think it is not perfect, it might last two years, do you say "That
patient is going to be all right for another two years" or do you
say, "It is only going to be all right for two years, I had better
put in a prosthesis now?"

BJORK: I would certainly not like to re-operate in two years.

YACOUB: I think the objective is to buy at least five years
if that is possible.

HILL: I do not think you can tell about this two years. My
experience of closed mitral valvotomy goes over 24 years and 800
cases. A high proportion of these now have valve replacements,
either at my hands or my registrar's hands, and I am particularly
struck by the description of the pathology of the valve and have
always been meticulous to describe all this in the operation note.
I agree that there are some whom you can tell will re-stenose
very rapidly, who will get stenosis below the valve. Equally
well, I have patients who had a severe valvar stenosis 20 years
ago who are still good functional results of a closed mitral
valvotomy. Rheumatic disease of the mitral valve is a progressive
process with a very variable rate. Some of them progress very
rapidly up to the time you operate on them and some very slowly
and go on slowly afterwards. Now, it is quite right to say that
the type of patient in this country has changed. In the first
10 or 14 years that I did mitral valvotomy the average age was
from about 18-25 and those were the patients who had their disability
from the mitral valve disease. The type of patient I am now asked
to operate on closed, because I have more experience than other
people in the hospital, are the patients of from 60-65. These are
the people who are getting their disability from the muscle
impaired by 60 years of rheumatic fever and not from the size of
the valve, and these people will get poorer results. This is an
entirely variable process, and I would like to know how you can
predict such a unique process. Equally well, I have a lot of
experience of mitral valvotomy where I have tried to repair the
mitral valve and I have come to the conclusion that in rheumatic

disease I am not going to know how to repair the mitral valve, and therefore, if I cannot get a successful mitral valvotomy, I will replace the valve.

CHAIRMAN: Well, perhaps the most difficult question is to know how long the mitral valve is going to stay open.

BJORK: No, I dare say that this was just guesswork. I am sure that if we get a certain amount of insufficiency and the patient is keeping a good blood pressure and so forth, I know that valve; it is just on the point of insufficiency. I cannot judge the re-stenosis, naturally, but I can judge that amount of insufficiency. I believe this patient has to be re-operated within a year or two. Guesswork, but some experience.

HILL: It is easy if it is a matter of mitral regurgitation. What I am worried about is this stenotic process. Most of us can assess the amount of regurgitation present at the end of an operation that will give a bad result in a few years.

CHAIRMAN: I am afraid nobody can answer that question unless someone from the audience wishes to volunteer.

BRAIMBRIDGE: I think there is just one thing, not quite answering the question but, I believe in my relatively experienced hands, that closed mitral valvotomy, the peanuts operation, can be done without prejudice to what you really are going to have to do perhaps eventually, which is a valve replacement. I have been doing, oddly enough, more closed mitral valvotomies because often, as Mr. Hill says, with a bad valve you get a surprisingly good result and if, in fact I am wrong and I get a bad result from a closed valvotomy then the open operation or valve replacement may come within a year. I do not consider that bad surgery. Every so often, as he says, one gets a remarkably good result. Closed mitral valvotomy does not really matter too much in the patient's history, because it does not prejudice the valve replacement in terms of second operation at all. I think this is a reasonable philosophy and the one I have come round to now.

YATES: Perhaps the discussion has gone on too long, but I really think it is going on because we have not really got the information to make a decision on the basic question. Each of us have our own ideas but the point is that the question will be answered when those performing open heart mitral valvotomy show the long-term results to be as good, or they must be better in fact, than the closed mitral valvotomy, and there is no way in which this question can be answered until that information is out.

CHAIRMAN: There is a tendency, when the heart is open, for the surgeons to appraise rather than take the extra time to see if he can reconstruct and that is always easier for the surgeon but not necessarily in the best interests of the patient.

ASHMORE: I would like to ask Mr. Braimbridge to elaborate on the problems of operating on patients with osteogenesis imperfecta.

BRAIMBRIDGE: The ones we have done have been a valve

replacement and a valvoplasty for mitral regurgitation in this condition. All I can say is that they have a haemmorhagic diathesis and in both these patients we had serious haemorrhagic problems and returned them to the theatre, and the tissues one was sewing in the heart and everywhere else were rather flimsy, though surprisingly you were not able to demonstrate any histological changes but, except for these two things, flimsy tissues and the tendency to bleed, they were the same as any other.

MEARNS: How bad a regurgitant situation can one accept after valvotomy?

YACOUB: The answer is that, with testing the valve, one does accept a localised very small amount of regurgitation - yes, and after operation approximately one quarter of the patients have a soft systolic murmur, so this is acceptable. Can I make another point regarding Mr. Yates' comments. I agree that we have not got the data. On the other hand I strongly disagree that you should compare the results of open and closed because the population of the patients is going to be different. You have to define the state of the valve in each group, very, very carefully, and then compare rather than say "a group of patients." It depends how you selected them.

SANDERSON: I wonder if Mr. Yacoub would mind describing his technique of decalcification?

YACOUB: This is calcium on the surface of the valve. It is extracted with a sharp instrument like one decalcifies the aortic root. If sometimes there are masses of calcium in the commissure, these are excised.

CHAIRMAN: Let us get on to mitral regurgitation. One of the questions I have is regarding the technique of plication of the redundant portion of the leaflet with ruptured chordae. I would like to ask Mr. Braimbridge if he does not feel that many of his patients also have a very dilated ring and need an annuloplasty done concurrently. They may have persistent mitral insufficiency although the redundant portion of the leaflet has been corrected.

BRAIMBRIDGE: Yes, sir, I am sure this is absolutely right but I think this is what taking 2cms of the ring at the back does. If one takes a parallelogram of cusp and ring out, rather than a cone as Dwight McGoon does, one is narrowing the ring by 2cm.

CHAIRMAN: In other words, you do your annuloplasty from the mid-portion of the posterior leaflet, whereas others have done it elsewhere.

BJORK: Well, I would just ask you if you are not more afraid of the circumflex artery if you tried to do an annuloplasty at the centre than if you did it by pushing up a third of the ring to the commissure?

BRAIMBRIDGE: We take a 3.0 Lembert suture in the valve ring at the mid-point of the posterior cusp and push the adjacent atrium under so that the suturing is then all superficial to the circumflex artery.

BLESOVSKY: I use the McGoon technique rather than the Gerbode technique and in the three cases I have done I have been satisfied with the result.

CHAIRMAN: Do you all agree with that on the panel? Mr. Braimbridge obviously does not because he does annuloplasty in a different place.

YACOUB: I am very similar to Mr. Braimbridge except that I excise that area and then these two points in the ring are really sutured together. There is no danger at all to the circumflex artery because you can see the fibrous attachment of the cusp.

CHAIRMAN: You said earlier that you also used this technique on the anterior leaflet, while Mr. Braimbridge does not. Can you clarify that difference?

YACOUB: Out of three patients with ruptured anterior cusp chordae I could excise the redundant bit and bring them together, rendering the valve competent.

BRAIMBRIDGE: And would you narrow the ring?

YACOUB: This time it is not extending right to the aortic root. It would be more of a wedge.

BJORK: How long did it hold up?

YACOUB: Over three years.

BJORK: Good.

ROSS: Sir, I am well aware of this floppy valve syndrome problem, as we all are, and the hugely dilated suddenly regurgitating valve. We are all happy to accept that it is a floppy valve or mucoid degeneration, but are you not just wondering why these cases occur at the age of three months, three years, eight years, that produce primary mitral regurgitation? I believe that there is a congenital basis; congenital clefts of the mitral valve. I know that Mr. Yacoub will perhaps disagree with it. If you study these redundant cusps carefully you will find that there is frequently a cleft to the posterior ring of the valve with its own commissural chordal attachment, and attached to its own papillary muscle. I find an increasing number of these patients are of a very young age and that, if you have a second development of something that will put up the left ventricular pressure, like aortic stenosis, hypertension in the older age group, and congenital deformity in the other age group, these then become important. I believe that these redundant valves are there from an early age. I would like to hear other peoples views on the congenital basis of this underlying pathology.

CHAIRMAN: How do members of the panel feel about this congenital theory as opposed to basic pathologic changes in the valve?

BRAIMBRIDGE: This does occur. I wonder if it is the same disease because a highly sensitised pathologist with whom I worked at St. George's has looked very carefully at a thousand consecutive post-mortems and has not found it in the young age group by the criteria described which may be different you see.

CARPENTIER: Can you tell me exactly where this cleft was?

ROSS: Exactly, yes.   (Draws on blackboard)

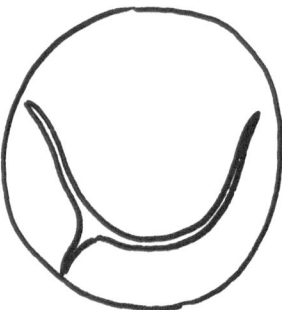

Figure 1.
Mitral Valve showing cleft in most characteristic site.

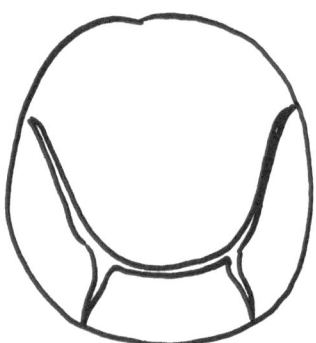

Figure 2.
Mitral Valve showing two clefts.

You will find a cleft characteristically there (Fig. 1) with a
cusp on either side of it with its own chordae, and commonly
secondly well developed here (Fig. 2).
    CARPENTIER: You never found one in the middle.
    ROSS: No, I mean yes.   You may think there is a cleft here.
In fact there is, but if you wanted to follow it right down to the
ring with its own chordal attachment, that is where I found it.
I am sure there can be one there but it is congenital.

CHAIRMAN: Does this cleft occur in Paris?

ROSS: Oh yes.

CARPENTIER: It is not different in Paris, it is different in the United States, because so few normal valves are examined. Those clefts are a normal variation.

ROSS: Normal variation?

CARPENTIER: Now just a moment. In a normal mural leaflet, in 10% of the cases, you have a cleft, you are right, but these clefts are normal. They are not the cause of regurgitation. It is a normal configuration.

ROSS: In 10% of the people?

CARPENTIER: In 10% of the cases. Well, that is my first point. Second point. You may have a larger leaflet than usual, I agree with that, but if this cleft - let us say it is normal - was the cause of regurgitation, you would have a localised lesion in this area.

ROSS: How do you explain it in a child of four, five or three?

CARPENTIER: You may be degenerate even at that age.

CHAIRMAN: In the absence of a pathologist no-one will answer this question. There are different causes of mitral insufficiency and perhaps primary rheumatic fever is the least common.

TURINA: I would just like to make a technical comment. Sometimes in Zurich we repair ruptured chordae by inserting a suture buttressed with Teflon felt through the cusp margin and the papillary muscle. Obviously you cannot tie the suture right down because it would produce regurgitation, but by injecting saline into the left ventricle you can tell how far to slide this suture down before you tie it. It does not always work, in about 12% we have to go to immediate valve replacement, but we have found it very useful in young patients.

MACARTNEY: It is worth mentioning that embyologically the mitral valve is originally quadricuspid and in 10% remains so.

CHAIRMAN: I would like you to try thinking about a question. There is another point concerning mitral valve disease that involves certain valves and that concerns the association of tricuspid insufficiency in the presence of significant mitral valve disease. As you know, there are those who favour doing notning to the insufficient tricuspid valve and those who favour reconstructing it - either with an annuloplasty or using Dr. Carpentier's ring, or in fact replacing it. How do you make this determination in such cases?

BRAIMBRIDGE: I used to use Dr. Carpentier's ring until it became a "Rolls-Royce" and was really as expensive as Professor Bjork's machine here, and I cannot afford to use it any more and have gone over, unfortunately for financial reasons, to the De Vager operation if there is any regurgitation now. I think the ultimate disaster in an operation is to go back on a patient who has had a mitral valve replacement and then develops progressive -

I do not understand why it is progressive - tricuspid regurgitation.
One has to do a median sternotomy with a paper thin right atrium
right under the sternum. I now think this is one of the ultimate
"bad news" operations, and I prefer to repair any tricuspid
regurgitation with the quick De Vager procedure at the time.

CHAIRMAN:. You would never leave a mild degree of tricuspid
insufficiency?

BRAIMBRIDGE: We have had four now who have gone on getting
progressively worse from what we assessed as haemodynamically
normal. I did not look at them but they felt normal, and have had
to re-operate. I have lost one case through opening the right
atrium with a median sternotomy.

CHAIRMAN: Is that the opinion of the rest of the panel?

BJORK: Yes, especially as in a careful follow-up investigation
it has been shown that practically all of the 20% that were not
improved had a progression of tricuspid incompetence. We as a
routine always make a right ventricular angiogram at the same run,
because we do an angiogram on all our cases and try to see tricuspid
regurgitation and find that there is a lot of them. If we see them
on an angiogram ahead of time we will certainly do this De Vager
procedure. Even for mild regurgitation we would like to do
annuloplasty at the first operation to avoid deterioration later on.

YACOUB: We find that the incidence of this severe tricuspid
regurgitation persisting after adequate mitral valve surgery is
very small indeed (2%).

GRAY: I would like to ask the surgeons about the redundant
cusp syndrome. Am I to understand that all the patients that I
see, and I see a lot of them, who have the mid-systolic click and
late systolic murmur, none of whom I have yet seen rupture a chorda,
are these all cases of the mucopolysaccharide infiltration, and
why do the ones that I see during their twenties, thirties, forties,
fifties, seem to live a normal life-span for the most part, whereas
if they have a progressive infiltration of the valve one would expect
them to do badly?

BRAIMBRIDGE: Until a chorda goes or a patient gets sub-acute
bacterial endocarditis, or has associated connective tissue disease,
statistically they are going to do well. They may have a little
noise but it is not going to be haemodynamically significant.

CHAIRMAN: Now we proceed to the last paper of the morning,
Professor Carpentier will discuss with us what we have already been
discussing today - treatment of mitral regurgitation.

Part II

PROJECTION OF
THE MYOCARDIUM

PROTECTION OF THE MYOCARDIUM DURING BYPASS BY LOCAL COOLING

ALAN K. YATES

CONSULTANT CARDIOTHORACIC SURGEON

GUY'S HOSPITAL, LONDON

Open heart operations are a compromise between cardiac access and an abnormal physiological state which places progressive stress on homeostasis and cell integrity. Cardiac arrest and especially atonic arrest greatly facilitates cardiac exposure and allows faster and more accurate manipulations of the heart. If a further acceptable compromise between the effect of myocardial ischaemia and accuracy and speed of operation can be delineated the total operative results should be further improved.

For over 20 years interest in, and the practice of myocardial arrest during open heart surgery has been applied. The methods used include:

1. Cardioplegia - using a chemically induced standstill.
2. Elective ventricular fibrillation.
3. Ischaemic arrest - which may be normothermic or hypothermic. If hypothermia is used this may be applied
   to the whole body or locally to the heart alone.

To summarise, the basic purpose of an arrested heart is to afford an easier operating environment to facilitate precise cardiac manipulation with shortening of the time taken for these manipulations. The fundamental problem is maintenance of the integrity of the myocardial intracellular enzyme systems. It is noted that even cardio-pulmonary bypass with a perfused beating heart is associated with gradual progressive intracellular decay of the myocardial enzyme system.

CONSIDERING ISCHAEMIC ARREST

In 1959 Shumway discussed the classification of elective
cardiac arrest for open heart surgery and subsequently developed
the regular use of a pericardial local myocardial cooling
technique. During the 1960s there was increasing use of normothermic ischaemic arrest periods, especially popularised by
Cooley et al (1966), and this was progressively extended up to
90 minutes (Reul et al. 1971). In this context the term normothermic
indicates bypass performed with no specific arrangements to produce
hypothermia by active cooling. It is common for the body temperature
to drift to levels of the order of 32°C.

Subsequently increasing awareness of myocardial damage due to
normothermic ischaemia occurred, and Reul and his associates (1971)
and Bloodwell's group (1969) described a relationship between
prolonged ischaemic arrest and low cardiac output syndrome post-
operatively. Reports by Miller (1964), Sato (1967), Mazza (1969),
Mundth (1970), Goldman (1971), Kirsch (1972), and MacGregor (1972),
with their associates and others, all indicate that the normothermic
ischaemic 'safe' time within which there is no significant functional
myocardial damage is of the order of 15 to 30 minutes. Beyond this
time there is increasingly significant irreversible changes of
mitochondrial fragmentation with breakdown of enzyme systems
involved in the Krebs cycle, which is the final aerobic phase for
the metabolism of glucose, amino acids and fatty acids (Gomes
et al. 1974). It is probably the increasing concentration of ammonia
in the myocardial cell, due to the inability to transport it or
break it down, that is the cause of protein destruction and the
observed irreversible changes (Kirsch et al. 1972). Ultra-microscopic
studies by Gomes et al. (1974) showed that after 30 minutes
normothermic ischaemia 47% of mitochondria show morphological
abnormalities, of which 13% were possibly significant.

At normothermia the myocardial metabolic rate continues at a
constant rate during an anoxic period (Gardner et al. 1971).
MacGregor et al. (1972), have shown that the safe period of
normothermic anoxic arrest is directly related to the metabolic
activity of the heart which in turn shows variation from patient
to patient (Gardner et al. 1971). This would explain the
considerable variation in myocardial response to normothermic
anoxia which is experienced clinically. In these experiments no
deaths occurred in any of the dogs whose hearts were exposed to
a normothermic anoxic period of 30 minutes or less, and it is
noted a significant number of dogs successfully withstood up to
60 minutes ischaemia.

The application of hypothermia will markedly reduce the
metabolic rate of the heart and increase the safety of ischaemic

arrest. Angell (1971) reporting a logarithmic relationship between
temperature and rate of anoxic myocardial damage. Oxygen demand
is reduced by 50% at a temperature of 28°C (Bigelow, 1958), and
myocardial anoxia is well tolerated for one hour in dogs at this
temperature. Analysis of mitochondrial enzyme integrity by
Gomes et al (1974), suggests that a myocardial temperature of not
greater than 20°C should be obtained for protection of one hour's
ischaemia.

The ideal hypothermic protection of ischaemic myocardium
would be a temperature of the order of 4°C-6°C. The cooling of
the myocardium should be uniform and quick, the oxygen tension in
myocardium dropping to zero within 10 minutes of aortic clamping
(Gardner et al. 1971), and any method should be easily applied
as an added complicated technique to gain a compromise situation
would not be accepted within an already complex operation. In
addition, the time spent in subsequently rewarming must not be
significantly long, as this would oppose the object of shortening
the manipulative time.

If a maximum ischaemic arrest time is decided upon which
answers the needs of all myocardial manipulations which would
benefit by arrest conditions, a modified hypothermia can be
accepted. Individual surgeons work at differing speeds and the
designated maximum ischaemic time must be an individual decision.
In considering this time factor it is important to realise that
the atonic non-perfused arrested heart affords markedly shortened
manipulative time compared to the time taken to perform the same
procedure in a perfused tonic heart.

In our unit our techniques indicate a need of one hour
maximum for any cardiac manipulations which would be significantly
aided by ischaemic arrest. From the evidence available, a
myocardial temperature of the order of 20°C would appear to offer
satisfactory myocardial protection for an ischaemic arrest of this
period of time.

CONSIDERING ISCHAEMIC ARREST WITH LOCAL HYPOTHERMIA

If only myocardial hypothermia is required it is unnecessary
to induce total body cooling as this involves significantly
longer time for the cooling and rewarming phases and also
markedly slows total body metabolism, rendering physiological
monitoring of the adequacy of bypass perfusion quality and
distribution more difficult.

Over a period of more than two years, all open heart
operations except the simplest and shortest, such as closure of
secundum atrial septal defects and pulmonary valvotomy, have been

performed with the aid of local hypothermic ischaemic arrest. In
a series of over 400 bypasses of all types we have exceeded the
maximum planned hypothermic ischaemic time of one hour on only one
occasion (1 hour, 12 minutes). This has resulted in definite
shortening of the operating time, great improvement in operating
conditions, and an objective improvement in overall results.

OUTLINE OF METHOD

When cardio-pulmonary bypass has been established, myocardial
cooling is instituted, after clamping the aorta and venting the
left heart, by rapidly filling the pericardial cavity with gravity
drip tubing fed normal saline, which has been cooled to a temperature
of $6^{\circ}C$-$10^{\circ}C$. The definitive cardiac procedure is immediately
proceeded with, and whenever cardiac incisions give access to
cardiac chambers these are also flush filled with the cold saline
solution. This is especially valuable in reference to the left
ventricular cavity. Initially the flushing rate is 500ml. of cold
solution over five minutes and subsequently 500ml. every 10-15
minutes throughout the cooling period. The intra-pericardial
cooling fluid level is kept as high as possible consistent with
the operative manipulations and the inflowing fluid is directed
over any part of the heart which is exposed above the fluid level.
The fluid level is maintained by sucking out the excess by a room
sucker, the tip of which is positioned at the back of the
pericardial space so that there is a good circulatory direction of
the cooling solution.

Myocardial temperatures obtained by this method were measured
by thermistor probes; one on the surface of the right ventricle
anteriorly; one on the surface of the left ventricle posteriorly
and a third introduced into the collapsed cavity of the left
ventricle via the left ventricular vent hole. In addition the
temperature of the posterior parietal pericardium was also measured.
All temperatures were measured at five minute intervals.

It was found that the posterior surface of the ventricular
mass had to be lifted off the posterior pericardium to allow free
circulation of the cooling solution over its surface. In addition
the proximity of the descending thoracic aorta to the posterior
pericardium resulted in a 'warm spot'. These two problems were
overcome by designing a double plate platform which is inserted
behind the heart (Fig. 1). The posterior plastic plate insulated
the warm area of the pericardium and the anterior fenestrated
steel plate allows free circulation of the cooling fluid round the
back of the heart, with good thermal conduction to the posterior
myocardium. If, in addition, a small sucker tip is fixed between
the plates at their edges the room sucker tubing can be attached
to it for controlled suction of cooling fluid. Left ventricular

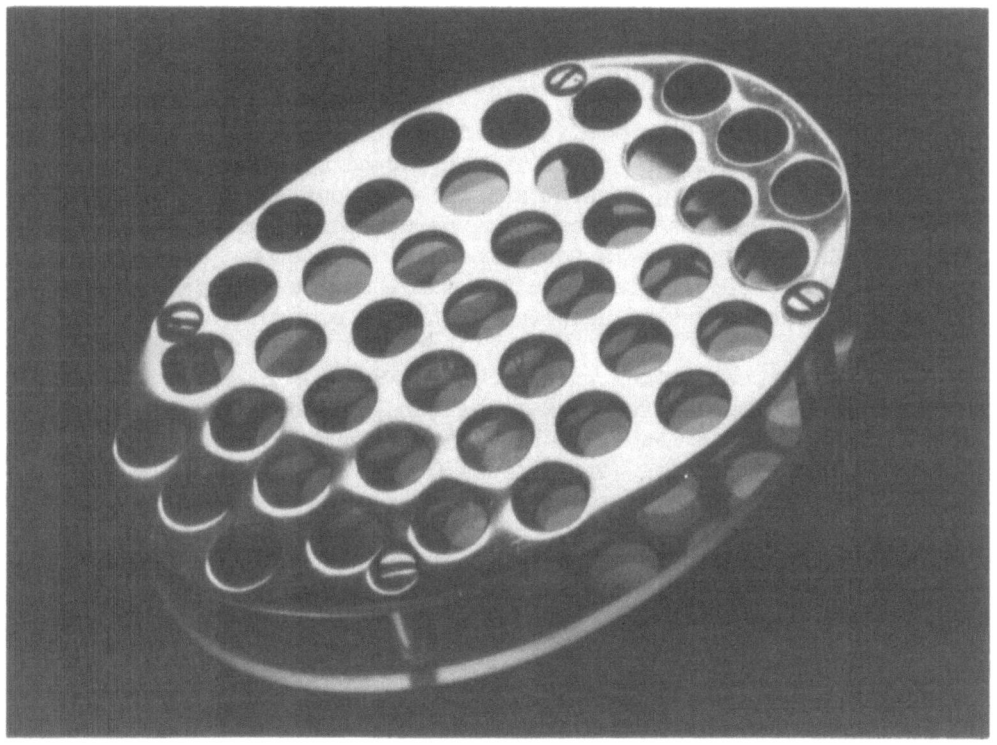

Figure 1

hypertrophy decreases the rate of cooling of the endocardial
surface and septum and it is important in these cases to
adequately flush-fill the left ventricular cavity with cooling
fluid at an early stage. It has been experimentally demonstrated
that hypertrophied myocardium undergoes more severe alterations
due to anoxic arrest than normal myocardium, (Levitsky et al 1971).
Significant left ventricular hypertrophy is fortunately usually
related to left ventricular outflow obstruction when the cavity
is easily accessible for cooling via the relevant cardiac incisions.

Pericardial cooling is continued throughout any period of
cardiac manipulations for which myocardial arrest is of advantage.
In all cases the cooling can be discontinued before the final
closure of cardiac incisions. This allows the myocardium to be
re-warmed by releasing the aortic clamp and bypass can be
discontinued in the usual manner at the end of the procedure with
no delay. Myocardial tone and contractility has been regained
within five minutes of re-warming in all cases.

To illustrate the experience in this procedure a series of 50 triple coronary artery bypass grafts are presented. Half of the cases were operated upon utilising local hypothermia with ischaemic arrest, and the other half were operated upon by maintaining myocardial perfusion with a non-clamped aorta. In this latter group normothermic ischaemic arrest was used for as short a time as possible whenever it was judged necessary for difficult coronary artery anastomoses to be adequately performed. These two series were not randomised, the non-cooled group being operated upon by a surgeon in the same unit who does not utilise hypothermic arrest but whose technique is otherwise comparable with my own. There were no hospital deaths in either group.

In the hypothermic ischaemic arrest group the total cardio-pulmonary bypass time varied between 1 hour 12 minutes, and 2 hours 1 minute, with a mean time of 1 hour 25 minutes; the hypothermic ischaemic time varied from 30 minutes to 51 minutes (mean time 40 minutes). In the normothermic group the total bypass time varied between 1 hour 58 minutes, and 2 hours 46 minutes with a mean time of 2 hours 12 minutes; the normothermic ischaemic time varied from 13 minutes to 60 minutes (mean time 24 minutes). (Table 1).

This confirms the significant saving factor of bypass time due to utilisation of planned hypothermic ischaemic arrest. It is important to note that the accepted safe ischaemic time is never exceeded in the hypothermic ischaemic group but is significantly exceeded in the normothermic group.

It can be concluded that difficult cases of triple coronary artery bypass grafts may require longer than a total of 30 minutes ischaemic arrest to gain satisfactory distal anastomoses.

Considering the cases which had pericardial cooling, Table 2 shows the details of body, myocardial and cooling fluid temperatures and left ventricular thickness. Table 3 shows a typical time related temperature curve of the myocardial and pericardial thermistor probes. It is seen the required cooling is satisfactorily rapidly gained and that warming is rapid at the end of the procedure. The higher temperatures in the noted ranges in Table 2 are the first temperatures measured at five minutes. These tables also illustrate the vulnerability of the endocardium and the posterior pericardial warm spot.

When used it is important that the procedure of local hypothermia is properly applied and that the cooling fluid is in fact at its expected temperature. If the cooling fluid has not reached 10°C or less, the system fails. The bottles of saline must be in the refrigerator for 12 hours before use and none must

TABLE I

Triple C.A.B.G. with local hypothermic ischaemic arrest
Bypass time: 1 hour 25 minutes (2.01 to 1.12)
Hypothermic ischaemic time: 40 minutes (30 to 51)

Triple C.A.B.G. with 'normothermic' conditions
Bypass time: 2 hours 12 minutes (2.46 to 1.58)
'Normothermic' ischaemic time: 24 minutes (13 to 60)

TABLE 2

PERICARDIAL COOLING

COOLING FLUID TEMP.	8 - 10°C
L.V. thickness	1.1 cm (0.9 to 1.5)
Cooling time	40 min (30 to 51)
Nasopharyngeal temp.	32.75°C (31.8 to 33.8)
Pericardial temp.	24.7°C (19.8 to 29.9)
Surface temp. R.V.	17.3°C (14.0 to 23.0)
Surface temp. L.V.	17.9°C (15.2 to 22.8)
L.V. cavity temp.	21.5°C (18.0 to 29.0)

TABLE 3

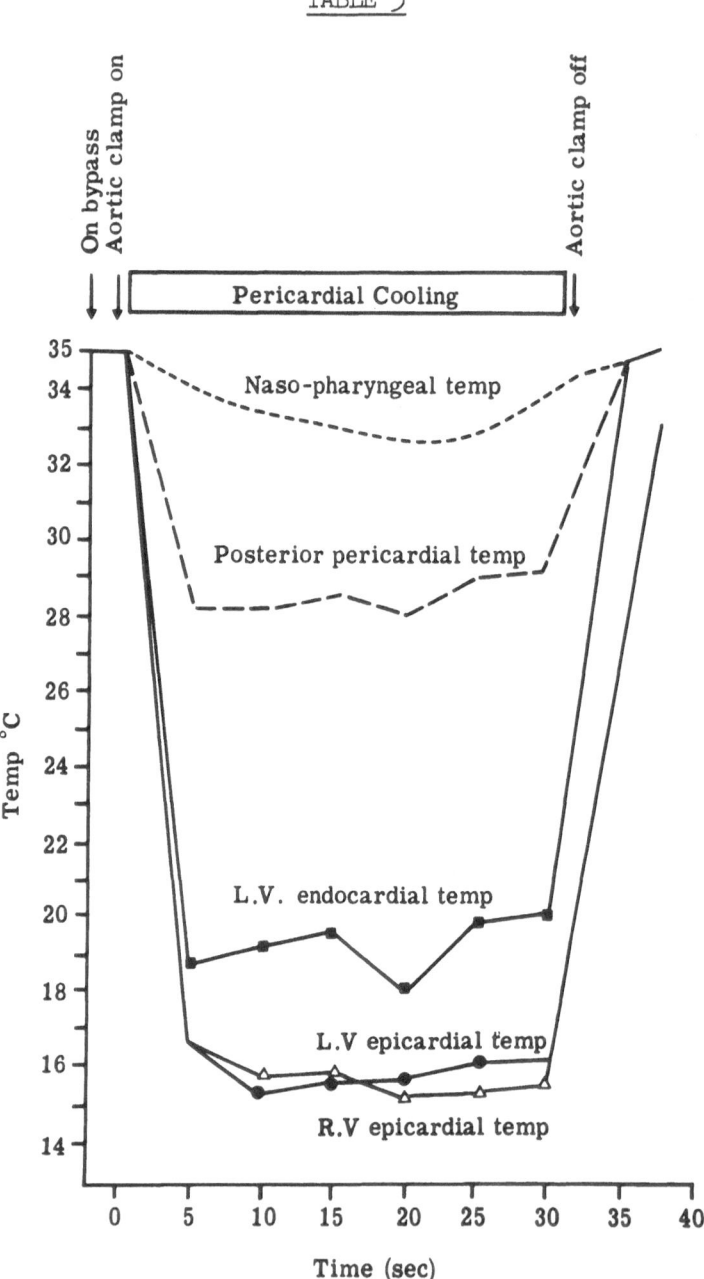

Table 4

PERICARDIAL COOLING

COOLING FLUID TEMP.	**11 - 20°·C**
L.V. thickness:	0.9 mm (0.8 to 1.2)
Cooling time:	41 min (30 to 55)
Nasopharyngeal temp.	33.1°C (31.6 to 34.8)
Pericardial temp.	25.6°C (24.8 to 28.0)
Surface temp.R.V.	20.0°C (16.2 to 24.0)
Surface temp.L.V.	22.2°C (18.6 to 24.6)
L.V. cavity temp.	28.3°C (27.0 to 29.8)

be removed or replaced by other than the person responsible for this part of the procedure. It is easily appreciated how bottles inadequately cooled may be used if this aspect is not tightly controlled. Table 4 illustrates a group of ten cases in which this happened. The special susceptibility to inadequate cooling by the left ventricular endocardium is clearly shown.

In summary we regularly use local hypothermic cardiac ischaemic arrest in all open heart operations except those of very short duration. The principle of this technique has been established over the years as a valid method by Shumway. It is very important for each surgeon to assess the required maximum time period of planned ischaemic arrest in relation to his own technique if a modified degree of hypothermia is to be used. It is suggested that one hours planned total ischaemic arrest is a reasonable time to allow all cardiac manipulations which benefit from a relaxed atonic heart. In triple valve replacement, for example, only the mitral and aortic replacement would be performed during hypothermic ischaemic arrest. The technique markedly improves operating conditions, and if correctly applied, significantly shortens operating time with no clinically recognised increase in myocardial morbidity or mortality.

REFERENCES

1. Angell, W.W. In discussion of (14)

2. Bigelow, W. G. (1958) Hypothermia. Surgery, 43:683.

3. Bloodwell, R.D., Kidd, J.N., Hallman, G.L., Buxdette, W.J., McMurtrey, M.J., and Cooley, D.A., (1969). Cardiac valve replacement without coronary perfusion. Clinical and laboratory observations in Brewer, L.A., III Editor. Prosthetic Heart Valves, Springfield, III. Charles C. Thomas, Publisher.

4. Cooley, D.A., Bloodwell, R.D., Beall, A.C., Gill, S.S., and Hallman, G.L., (1966). Total cardiac valve replacement using SCDK-Cutter Prosthesis: Experience with 250 consecutive patients. Ann.Surg.,164:429.

5. Gardner, T.J., Brantigan, J.W., Perna, A.M., Bender, H.W., Bramley, R.K., and Gott, V.L., (1971). Intramyocardial gas tensions in the human heart during coronary artery - Saphenous vein bypass. J.Thorac.Cardiovasc.Surg., 62:844.

6. Goldman, B.S., Trimble, A.S., Sherverini, M.A., Teasdale, S.L., Silver, M.D., and Elliot, G.E. (1971). Functional and metabolic effects of anoxic cardiac arrest. Ann.Thorac.Surg, 11:122.

7. Gomes, O.M., Pedroso, F.I., Pereira, S.N., Ayoub, A.H., Kwang, W.T., Bittencourt, D., and Zerbim, E.J. (1974). Mitochondrial enzymatic alterations produced in the myocardium by anoxic cardiac arrest. J.Thorac.Cardiovasc.Surg., 67:649.

8. Kirsch, U., Rodewald, G., and Kalmar, P. (1972). Induced ischaemic arrest: Clinical experience with Cardioplegia in open heart surgery. J.Thorac. Cardiovasc.Surg., 63:121.

9. Levitsky, S., Sloane, R.E., Mullin, E.M., McIntosh, C.L., and Morrow, A.G., (1971). Normothermic myocardial anoxia. Effects on the canine heart with left ventricular outflow obstruction. Ann.Thorac.Surg., 11:229.

10. MacGregor, D.C., Mehta, V.S., Metric, F.N., Krajicek, M., Kryspin, J., Botz, C.C., and Trimble, A.S.(1972). Normothermic anoxic arrest of the heart. Is there a means of estimating the safe period? J.Thorac.Cardiovasc.Surg., 64:833.

11. Mazza, L.V., Anversa, P., Morgutti, L., and Taso, A. (1969). Changes of the myocardial ultrastructure during open heart

surgery with extracorporeal circulation. J.Cardiovasc.Surg.
10;212.

12. Miller, D.R., Rasmussen, P., and Klionsky, B. (1964).
Reversibility of morphologic changes following elective
cardiac arrest. Ann.Surg., 159:205.

13. Mundth, E.D., Sokol, D.M., Levine, F.H., and Austen, W.G.
(1970). Evaluation of methods for myocardial protection
during extended periods of aortic cross-clamping and hyposic
cardia c arrest. Bull.Soc.Int.Chir., 29:227.

14. Reul, G.J., Morris, G.C., Jr., Howell, J.F., Crawford, E.S.,
Sandiford, F.M., and Sukasch, D.C. (1971). The safety of
ischaemic cardiac arrest in distal coronary artery bypass.
J.Thorac.Cardiovasc.Surg., 62:511.

15. Sato, R., Ogawa, K., Okada, M., Takeda, Y., and Kumira, K
(1967). Studies on the maximal time limit for total
occlusion of the coronary circulation by determination of
the enzymatic activity level in blood. J.Thorac.Cardiovasc.
Surg., 53:231.

16. Shumway, N.E. (1959). A classification of elective cardiac
arrest for open heart surgery. Dis.Chest, 36:315-8.

PROTECTION OF THE MYOCARDIUM BY CORONARY PERFUSION

G. M. REES

CONSULTANT CARDIOTHORACIC SURGEON

ST. BARTHOLOMEW'S HOSPITAL, LONDON, EC1

Some myocardial damage is probably an inevitable result of open heart surgery and its extent may profoundly influence both the early and late morbidity and mortality. Apart from relatively crude survival data, there are several more sophisticated techniques available for assessing myocardial changes. These include electron microscopy and the measurement of alterations in myocardial metabolism and cardiac performance.

The use of such methods has led to the identification of the main factors liable to cause myocardial damage. In addition, the instigation of techniques designed specifically to protect the myocardium from damage can be evaluated with their use. We have applied the experience gained from these data to isolated mitral valve replacement in man in which the myocardium is protected by coronary perfusion using aortic root cannulation.

SITES OF MYOCARDIAL DAMAGE

Histological changes are demonstrable in the myocardium within 15-20 mins. of the cessation of coronary perfusion at normothermia (Burdette & Ashford, 1965). These are easily seen by electron microscopy. The early changes occur in the mitochondria, which show diminution in number and size of coarse granules, condensation of the inner membrane and general swelling. The nuclear chromatin shows marginal clumping. After 45 mins. of ischaemia, swelling and vacuolization of the mitochondria with disruption of their christae and membranes occurs. However, the contractile elements are considerably more resistant, although separation of myofibrillary bundles is apparent at 30 mins. Because mitochondria are

particularly abundant in cardiac muscle and are the site of action
of the Krebs cycle, terminal electron transport and oxidative
phosphorylation damage may result in severe biochemical disturbances.

METHODS OF ASSESSING MYOCARDIAL DAMAGE

Anaerobic metabolism is followed by biochemical changes which
are readily detectable in coronary sinus blood. These include
changes in lactate and enzyme production and efflux of electrolytes,
particularly potassium from intracellular sources. Additional
stimuli, for example anoxia and induced ventricular fibrillation,
may cause a change in total blood flow as well as redistribution
of blood within the heart.

Cardiac performance may be calculated after various manoeuvres
and repeated determinations have been made in the recovery phase.

NORMOTHERMIC ISCHAEMIC ARREST

The length of time that the heart can tolerate ischaemia at
normothermia without sustaining permanent damage is a matter of
considerable debate. Undoubtedly the main advantage of this
commonly employed technique is that the surgical field is both
bloodless and flaccid. However, it has been criticised and
implicated in the pathogenesis of both low post-operative cardiac
output and more importantly in the production of permanent
myocardial damage.

Stemmer and his colleagues (1973) showed that the survival
rate in normal dogs undergoing normothermic ischaemic arrest on
bypass was diminished and also that the cardiac output in those
recovering was significantly lower than in the controls.
However, the duration of ischaemia was long (1-2 hours) and is
therefore not directly comparable to the clinical situation where
the heart is abnormal and the aortic cross-clamping time is less.

Nevertheless, a delay of 15 mins. in commencing coronary
perfusion in man undoubtedly produces abnormalities in both
lactate and oxygen metabolism (Ison et al, 1973), suggesting that
the length of ischaemia tolerated by the pathological heart is
very small.

Similarly the use of intermittent perfusion is far from
satisfactory. Studies in normal pigs have shown that three
periods of intermittent ischaemia (30 mins.) with intervening
periods of coronary perfusion (5 mins.) caused marked redistribution
of blood away from the sub-endocardium (Engleman et al, 1975), and
although shortening of the ischaemic period to 15 mins. diminished
this effect, it was still present.

VENTRICULAR FIBRILLATION

The normal heart is an unsatisfactory model for comparison with the pathological human heart. This led Buckberg and colleagues to investigate functional and metabolic changes following ventricular fibrillation in both the normal and hypertrophied heart (Hottenrott et al, 1973).

Spontaneous ventricular fibrillation in the normal dog heart is followed by marked increase in both oxygen consumption and coronary blood flow, the latter being particularly apparent in the subendocardial region. However, in dogs with left ventricular hypertrophy (previously produced by aortic constriction), ventricular fibrillation produced a different response. Neither total coronary flow nor myocardial oxygen consumption was found to increase, nor was the flow of blood to the subendocardial zone increased. Metabolic changes were also different in normal and hypertrophied hearts. Ventricular fibrillation of 60 minutes duration in the normal heart caused no detectable abnormality, whereas in the hypertrophied heart, marked lactate production and potassium efflux occurred. The latter also showed considerable depression of myocardial performance after bypass compared with normal hearts. Additionally, fibrillated hypertrophied hearts showed histological damage in the subendocardial region.

A similar response has been described following the application of a fibrillating current to the hypertrophied pig heart (Becker et al, 1973) which is of particular interest since considerable anatomical similarities exist between the human and porcine coronary circulations.

In man the ventricle consumes as much oxygen when fibrillating as during regular contraction whilst enzyme levels are persistently raised following restoration of sinus rhythm, indicating intra-operative myocardial damage (Ison et al, 1973).

METHODS OF PROTECTING THE MYOCARDIUM

i) Hypothermia. The use of deep hypothermia applied either topically (Griepp et al, 1973; Stemmer et al, 1973; McCallister et al, 1975) or by whole body perfusion (Keen et al, 1970) provides considerable myocardial protection from ischaemia. Mitochondrial abnormalities undoubtedly occur but are less marked than at normothermia and are compatible with post-operative survival in both man and experimental animals.

ii) Coronary Perfusion. Although intraoperative coronary perfusion is undeniably "unphysiological" there is considerable evidence that it is the best method of myocardial protection. Most of its disadvantages are related to the difficulties of

coronary cannulation and the possible damage which may result
(Griepp et al, 1973; Robicsek et al, 1970). In Stemmer's
experiments on normal dogs, the best results, in terms of overall
survival, post-operative cardiac performance and histopathological
changes, were obtained when the coronaries were perfused with
hypothermic blood. Those receiving topical hypothermia with
ischaemia did not do so well (Stemmer et al, 1973). Myocardial
metabolism is more satisfactory if the heart is allowed to beat
in sinus rhythm (Ison, 1973). However, coronary flow rates should
be less than 300 ml/min. since higher flow rates produce raised
levels of creatine phosphokinase, lactic dehydrogenase and SGOT
in coronary sinus blood. Subendocardial perfusion is particularly
well maintained in sinus rhythm (Becker et al, 1973).

Coronary perfusion has also been compared with whole body
hypothermia as a method of protecting the myocardium during aortic
valve replacement in man (Sapsford et al, 1973). Cardiac
performance, metabolism and isoenzyme release did not differ in
the two groups. However, bypass and aortic cross-clamp time were
reduced by 21% and 27% respectively in the hypothermic group and
70% in this group had evidence of myocardial damage and 26% had
electrocardiographic changes of either infarction or ischaemia.
However, the short duration of perfusion at low temperatures
raises doubts concerning the efficacy of cardiac cooling. This
work does not provide data on the value of topical hypothermia.

A comparison of metabolic activity between hearts perfused
at normothermia ($36^{\circ}C$) and mild hypothermia ($30^{\circ}C$) did not reveal
detectable differences in acid/base measurements, electrolytes
or the formation of energy-producing substrates (Moffitt et al,
1971). As might be anticipated, oxygen consumption was threefold
in the normothermic heart.

Thus, there is good evidence that even short periods of
ischaemia at normothermia have deleterious effects on the heart.
Although ventricular fibrillation may facilitate the surgical
technique, harmful effects may occur, particularly in the
subendocardial region of the hypertrophied heart.

Aortic root perfusion is particularly suitable for mitral
valve replacement because damage to the main coronary arteries
is avoided. This technique was introduced to St. Bartholomew's
Hospital in 1974.

METHODS

The aorta is cannulated above and below the aortic ·cross-
clamp which prevents systemic air embolization. This is an
undoubted hazard and occurs when the heart is allowed to beat and

reliance is placed on the vent for prevention of ejection into the aorta. Initially most cases were done at normothermia although recently the patients have been cooled to 30°. This slows the heart rate and decreases contractility thus making the operation technically easier. Aortic root flow is kept below 300 ml/min, the pressure being kept at about 70 mm/Hg. The left ventricle is vented via the apex and can generally cope if mild aortic regurgitation is present. A small left atrium tends to increase the difficulties but not unduly. Occasionally transient induced ventricular fibrillation is used while the valve is tied down. Otherwise if ventricular fibrillation occurs during the operation, it is corrected immediately. An interrupted suture technique is employed throughout.

Fifty-one patients have undergone mitral valve replacement using this technique. Thirty-eight were female and thirteen male. Their ages ranged from 20-68 (mean 50 years). Twenty-three (47%) had previously had mitral valve surgery: in most this was closed-mitral valve surgery, in some on more than one occasion.

Pulmonary vascular resistance (PVR) was determined in 44. In 32 PVR was between one and five units; in nine between five and ten units and in three, in excess of ten units. Seven had aortic regurgitation but of insufficient severity to warrant aortic valve replacement.

RESULTS

There was one hospital death in this series. She died of completely unexpected cardiac arrest during an otherwise apparently uneventful post-operative recovery, two weeks after operation.

The group as a whole were remarkable for the ease with which they were weaned from bypass and the rapidity with which they passed through the recovery room to the post-operative ward.

Three patients developed paravalvar leak and required reoperation. One patient early in the series underwent reoperation without coronary perfusion. She died in the operating room. Two others were reoperated using coronary perfusion and made uneventful recoveries.

No neurological abnormalities occurred in this group and is attributed to the fact that ejection of air into the aorta cannot occur during the valve replacement and to the care taken to evacuate all air prior to release of aortic clamp at the end.

Although regurgitation through an incompetent aortic valve prevents accurate measurement of coronary flow, it is reasonable to infer that coronary perfusion is adequate, provided the heart continues in sinus rhythm without the development of electrocardiographic changes of ischaemia. Mild hypothermia in such cases increases the safety margin and is advised.

CONCLUSIONS

Extensive clinical and experimental data indicate that myocardial damage occurs during open heart operations. Effective methods of myocardial protection are now available and their efficacy is confirmed in the series of patients undergoing mitral valve replacement reported here. Damage to the main coronary arteries can be avoided by aortic root cannulation while possible damage to the small coronary vessels is avoided by careful control of perfusion pressure and flow rates.

The technical difficulties of surgery are not increased by this method. For example, access is not significantly impeded by the aortic root since this is not particularly tense and aortic regurgitation is generally well controlled by left ventricular vent suction.

Three patients developed paravalvar leaks early in the series but this has not been seen recently. This improvement is probably due to deeper placement of interrupted sutures and the use of a short period of ventricular fibrillation while the sutures are tied down.

REFERENCES

Becker, R., Shizgal, H., Dobell, A.: Distribution of coronary blood flow during cardiopulmonary bypass in pigs. Annals of Thoracic Surgery, 16, 228-238, 1973.

Benzing, G., Stockerty, J., Nave, E., Kaplan, S.: Intermittent myocardial ischaemia during cardiopulmonary bypass. Journal of Thoracic and Cardiovascular Surgery, 65, 108-111, 1973.

Burdette, W. J., and Ashford, T. P.,: Structural changes in the human myocardium following hypoxia. Journal of Thoracic and Cardiovascular Surgery, 50, 210-220, 1965.

Englemann, R., Adler, S., Gouge, T.: The effect of normothermic anoxic arrest and ventricular fibrillation on the coronary blood flow distribution of the pig. Journal of Thoracic and Cardiovascular Surgery, 69, 858-869, 1975.

Griepp, R., Stinson, E.B., Shumway, N.E.: Profound local hypothermia for myocardial protection during open heart surgery. Journal of

Thoracic and Cardiovascular Surgery, 66, 731-741, 1973.

Hottenrott, C.E., Towers, B., Kurkji, H.J., Maloney, J.V., Buckberg, G.: The Hazard of ventricular fibrillation in hypertrophied ventricles during cardiopulmonary bypass. Journal of Thoracic and Cardiovascular Surgery, 66, 742-753, 1973.

Isom, O.W., Kutin, N.D., Falk, E.A., Spencer, F.C.: Patterns of myocardial metabolism during cardiopulmonary bypass and coronary perfusion. Journal of Thoracic and Cardiovascular Surgery, 66, 705-721, 1973.

Keen, G., Dowlatshahi, K.: The effects of circulatory arrest during profound hypothermia upon human myocardial fine structure. Cardiovascular Research, 4, 348-354, 1970.

McCallister, L.P., Munger, B.L., Tyers, G., Hughes, H.C.: The effect of different methods of protecting the myocardium on lysosomal activation and acid phosphatase activity in the dog heart after one hour bypass. Annals of Thoracic Surgery, 69, 644-663, 1975.

Moffitt, E.A., Sessler, A.D., Molnar, G.D., McGoon, D.C. Normothermia versus hypothermia for whole body perfusion: effects on myocardial and body metabolism. Anaesthesia and analgesia, 50, 505-516, 1971.

Robicsek, F., Tam, W., Daugherty, H., Mullen, D.: Myocardial protection during open heart surgery. Annals of Thoracic Surgery, 10, 340-353, 1970.

Sapsford, R., Blackstone, E.H., Kirklin, J.W., Karp, R.B., Kouchoukos, N.: Coronary perfusion versus cold ischaemic arrest during aortic valve surgery. Circulation, 49, 1190-1199, 1974.

Stemmer, E., McCart, P., Stanton, W., Thibault, W., Dearden, L., Connolly, J.: Functional and Structural alteration in the myocardium during aortic cross-clamping. Journal of Thoracic and Cardiovascular Surgery, 66, 754-770, 1973.

CONTRIBUTION TO DISCUSSION ON MYOCARDIAL PRESERVATION

T. A. H. ENGLISH

PAPWORTH HOSPITAL, CAMBRIDGE

Mr. Chairman, at the beginning of this afternoon's symposium you said you were primarily interested in hearing about methods of myocardial preservation that were applicable to most operative situations. I would like to describe a method of selective cardiac hypothermia without coronary perfusion which fulfils this criterion in that we use it for all open heart operations that are judged to require more than 15 minutes aortic cross-clamping.

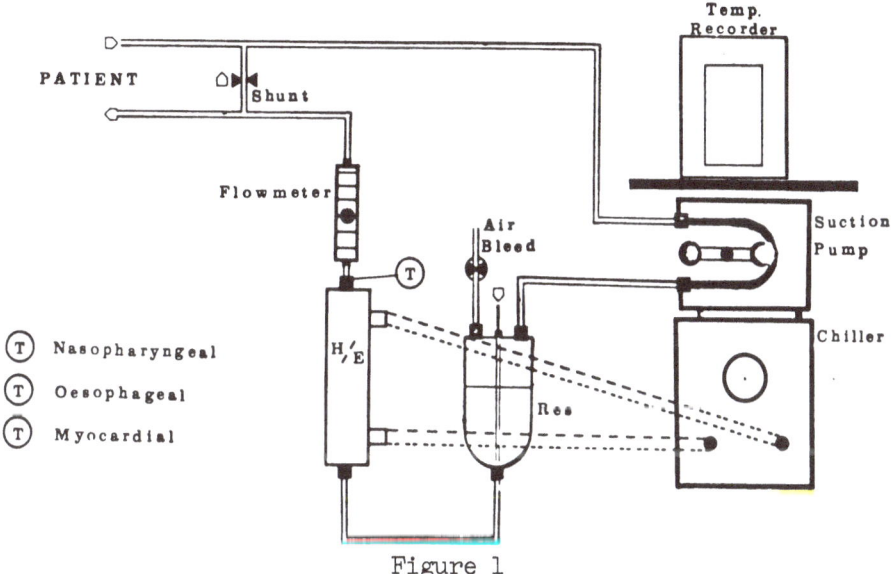

Figure 1

Recirculation Circuit for Selective Cardiac Hypothermia

When we first considered using topical hypothermia we rec-
ognized that the single most important requirement was to ensure
rapid and uniform cooling of the heart to a temperature at which
metabolism becomes almost negligible. To this end we designed a
simple recirculation cooling circuit capable of delivering up to
600 ml. per minute of fluid into the pericardium at 4°C.

Fluid is aspirated from the pericardial cavity by a Sarns
pump that circulates it through a reservoir and heat-exchanger
and then returns the cooled fluid to the pericardium. A temperature recorder, mounted on the trolley, monitors the myocardial
temperature continuously, and the flow rate of the cooling fluid
is also measured. Advantages of the system include rapid cooling
of the myocardium, flexibility of myocardial temperature control,
and simplicity of operation.

Figure 2 illustrates the continuous nasopharyngeal and
myocardial temperatures recorded during aortic valve replacement.

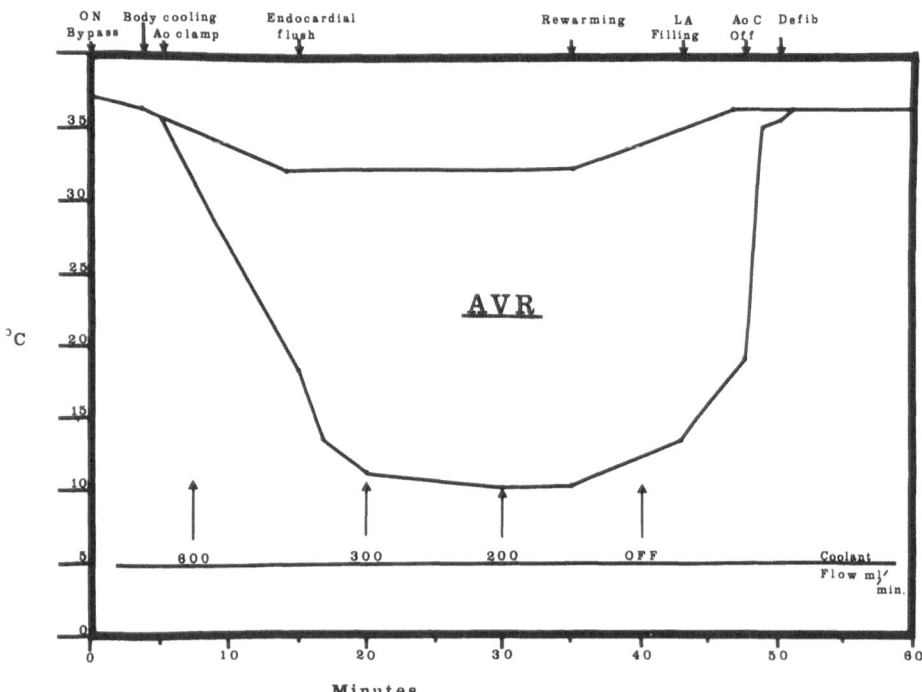

Fig. 2. Continuous Nasopharyngeal and Myocardial temperatures
during Aortic Valve Replacement

Pericardial cooling is commenced shortly after the aorta is clamped and the endocardial surface of the left ventricle is flushed with cold fluid (we use Hartmann's solution) as soon as the valve is excised. In this way the myocardial temperature is reduced to 15°C. within twelve minutes of aortic clamping.

Figure 3 is a similar record obtained during mitral valve replacement. Complete immersion of the ventricles is not poss-ible during this procedure because of the posteriorly situated left atriotomy. The aortic root is therefore flushed with 500 ml. Hartmann's solution at 4°C. as soon as the aorta has been clamped to provide rapid initial cooling of the myocardium. This fluid is aspirated via a cardiotomy sucker held in the left atrium and forms part of the "pump prime". The table is then rotated 20° to the left and pericardial cooling commenced, allowing the fluid level to rise just below the level of the left atriotomy.

We use mild systemic hypothermia to diminish the rewarming effect of bronchial return to the left side of the heart.

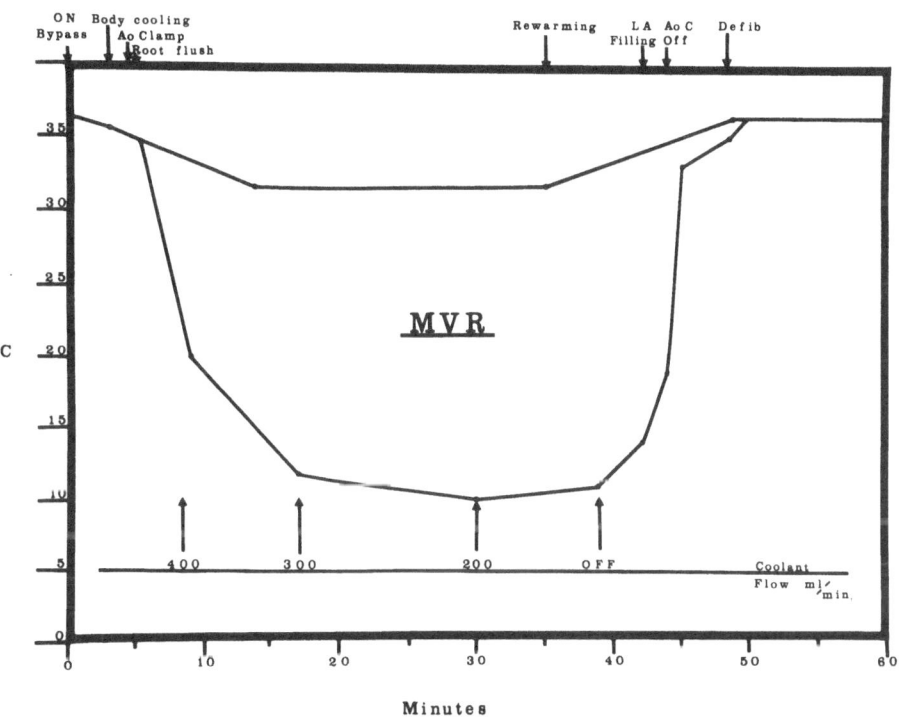

Fig. 3. Continuous Nasopharyngeal and Myocardial temperatures during Mitral Valve Replacement

Systemic rewarming is instituted ten minutes before the aortic
clamp is due to be released, after which myocardial rewarming
takes place rapidly. Defibrillation is usually accomplished
within three minutes of re-establishing coronary perfusion and
a period of at least ten minutes supportive perfusion is then
always allowed before cardiopulmonary bypass is discontinued.

We have recently analysed the first one hundred operations
in which this system of myocardial preservation was used.
Details of these operations are presented in Table I.

TABLE I

		OPERATIONS		MORTALITY	
		Redo	E	Hospital	Late
A.V.R.*	60	8	5	1 (9 days)	2
Congenital	19	4	-	-	-
M.V.R.	12	1	-	1 (48 days)	1
M.V.R. + A.V.R.+	7	3	-	-	-
Miscellaneous	2	1	1	-	-
	100	17	6	2%	3%

```
*   3 had replacement ascending aorta
+   1 had replacement ascending aorta
E = Emergency
```

You will note that seventeen patients had previous open
intracardiac procedures and that there were six emergency operations. The duration of cardiac ischaemia varied from 20 to 153
minutes with a mean of 72 minutes. Myocardial temperature during
ischaemia averaged 16°C. There were two hospital deaths, one at
9 days and one at 48 days, and two late deaths. An analysis of
postoperative electrocardiographic changes compares favourably
with standard techniques using coronary perfusion.

Table II lists the operations performed for congenital heart disease. We believe the method is particularly suitable for this type of surgery as good immersion of the heart can usually be obtained and also excellent operating conditions are provided.

TABLE II

CONGENITAL OPERATIONS

Fallot's tetralogy*	10
Aortic stenosis (2 subvalvar; 1 supravalvar)	3
V.S.D.	2
D.O.R.V. with d-malposition and P.S.	1
"Corrected" T.G.A. with V.S.D. and P.S.	1
R.V. infundibular resection (redo)	1
Partial anomalous P.V.D.	1
	19

* 5 had reconstruction of outflow tract
  2 with homografts.

In conclusion I believe that this method of selective cardiac hypothermia offers the following advantages:-

1. Satisfactory preservation of the heart during anoxic arrest.

2. Protection of the coronary vasculature from microembolism.

3. No problems with or as a result of selective coronary perfusion.

4. Less damage to platelets and other blood constituents because of less coronary suction.

5. It provides a quiet, relaxed and bloodless field which offers perfect conditions for accurate surgical repair.

METABOLIC PROTECTION DURING ISCHEMIC CARDIAC ARREST

M. V. BRAIMBRIDGE, D. J. HEARSE, D. A. STEWART

THE MYOCARDIAL METABOLISM LABORATORIES, THE RAYNE

INSTITUTE, ST. THOMAS HOSPITAL, LONDON

Open heart surgery requires ideally a still and relaxed heart. Cardiac arrest in diastole can be induced by several procedures (1-10) which may or may not involve coronary perfusion. Clearly coronary perfusion throughout the period of arrest is ideal but the simplicity and practical advantages of ischemic arrest have resulted in its widespread use (7,8). However, the use of ischemic arrest has been criticised (1,11,12,13) because, associated with its prolonged use is the onset of irreversible metabolic and ultrastructural damage. The important question therefore arises:- is there any way in which the ischemic period can be extended or the onset of irreversible damage be reduced or delayed?

Immediately following the onset of ischemia a number of functional, metabolic and morphological changes occur (14). These changes are initially of a reversible nature and if blood flow is restored to the ischemic tissue during this phase there is complete resumption of normal metabolism and function. If ischemia is maintained for longer periods irreversible damage occurs, the restoration of blood flow no longer consistently reverses the injury and permanent impairment of functional capacity occurs. The time taken for the onset of irreversible damage is determined by a number of factors such as the severity of ischemia; the nutritional, hormonal and contractile status of the myocardium; the availability of energy supplies such as glycogen, adenosine triphosphate (ATP) and creatine phosphate (CP); the metabolic capacity for anaerobic energy production; the age and temperature of the myocardium and the composition of the coronary blood in the tissues at the onset of ischemia.

Altering the temperature of the myocardium and the composition of the extra-cellular fluid provides an effective means of modifying the rate at which ischemic tissue deteriorates. The use of topical hypothermia and the consequent reduction of metabolic rate affords considerable protection to the ischemic myocardium (2,4,9,15,16, 17,18). Similarly, the pioneering work of Bretschneider (19) and Kirsch (20,21) and their colleagues has emphasised the value of the infusion of various cardioplegic and protective solutions into the coronary circulation just prior to ischemia.

The objective of the studies reported in this paper was to use the isolated rat heart to search for and individually assess the potential protective value of a variety of agents which could be combined on a rational basis to form a solution which, if infused into the coronary bed prior to ischemia, could combat the deleterious changes induced by ischemia and thereby afford protection to the myocardium. The requirements of such a solution were that it should arrest the heart rapidly in diastole, be non-toxic and also be freely and rapidly reversible on reperfusion. In addition to its cardioplegic action it was hoped that such a solution would also minimise ischemic changes such as acidosis, cell swelling, depletion of energy reserves, loss of ions, metabolic disruption and the occurrence of dysrhythmias.

METHODS

Male rats (300g) of the Sprague Dawley strain were used and the perfusion techniques were as described previously (2,22). The perfusion circuit is illustrated in Figure 1. The perfusion fluid (gassed with 95% O_2+5% CO_2) was Krebs-Henseleit bicarbonate buffer pH 7.4 (24) which during all working periods contained 11mmol glucose. The same buffer, without glucose but with various additives, was used for coronary infusion. The experimental time course is illustrated in Figure 2. The heart is subjected to an initial period of aerobic perfusion; it is then bypassed, subjected to two minutes of coronary infusion and then a period of ischemia. After the ischemic period the heart is reperfused and the functional recovery over a 20 minute period is monitored and expressed as a percentage of the initially obtained control value. In this way the recovery of the heart can be related to the nature of the infusate and the duration of ischemia.

RESULTS

In initial experiments a base line for ischemia damage was obtained. Hearts (n=6) were infused for two minutes prior to ischemia with substrate-free Krebs bicarbonate buffer. In this way no nutrients or protective agents were present in the vascular fluid during the ischemic period. Under these conditions,

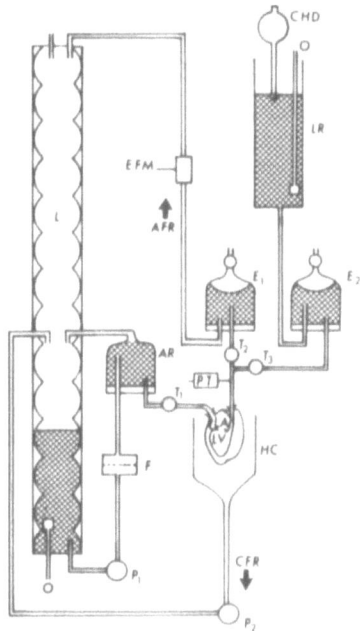

Figure 1

Perfusion Circuit: Following excision of the heart, the aorta
and left atrium were cannulated to produce a working heart
preparation (22). The heart was maintained in a thermostatically
controlled chamber (HC) which (with the exception of topical
hypothermia experiments) was maintained at 37°C. In the working
model, taps T_1 and T_2 were open, and perfusion fluid entered the
heart via the left atrium (LA) from a reservoir (AR) located 20cm
above the heart. The left ventricle (LV) ejected perfusate via
the aorta and an eleasticity chamber (E_1) against a 100cm
hydrostatic pressure to the top of the lung (L). An electro-
magnetic flowmeter (EMF) continuously recorded the aortic flow
rate (AFR). The perfusion fluid was reoxygenated in the
thermostatically maintained lung (37°C) and returned via a
peristaltic pump (P_1) and a cellulose acetate filter (F) to the
atrial reservoir (AR) which was thus maintained at a constant
head. The coronary perfusate exited into the heart chamber (HC)
and was returned via a peristaltic pump (P_2) to the lung for
reoxygenation (O). The coronary flow rate (CFR) could be monitored.
Aortic pressure was monitored by a pressure transducer (PT).
Simulated bypass was achieved by closing taps T_1 and T_2. Coronary
infusion was achieved by opening tap 3 and oxygenated (O) infusion
fluid flowed from a reservoir (LR) and constant head device (CHD)
via an elasticity chamber (E_2) to a side arm of the aortic cannula.
This essentially represented a Langendorff (23) retrograde
perfusion.

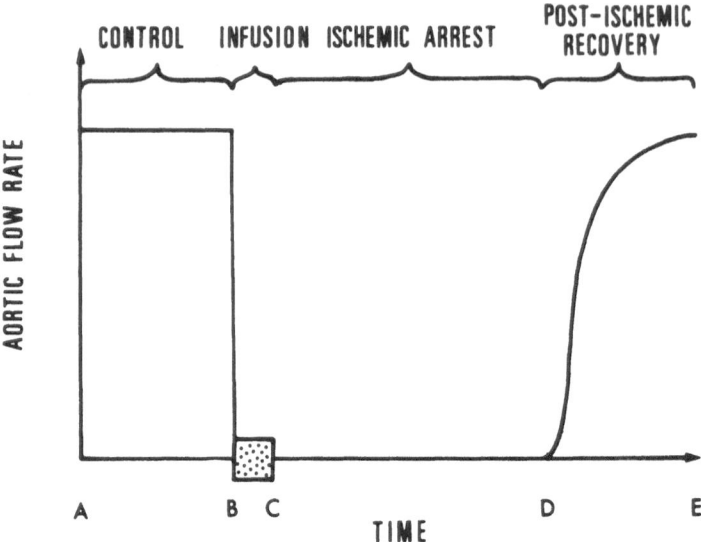

Figure 2

Experimental Time Course: At point A the heart is mounted on the
apparatus and is subjected to aerobic perfusion. Between A and B
there is a 20 minute control period during which time control
values for aortic flow, coronary flow, heart rate, ventricular
pressure and other parameters of cardiac function can be obtained.
At time B the heart is bypassed by clamping the aortic and left
atrial cannulae. Under these conditions, aortic flow, as shown
in this figure, falls to zero. For two minutes between B and C
the coronary system is infused via the root of the aorta with the
solution of choice. At time C infusion is terminated and between
C and D the heart is ischemic. At time D the aortic and left
atrial cannulae are unclamped, atrial perfusion is resumed and
the recovery of the heart is monitored between D and E.

hearts subjected to 30 minutes ischemia totally failed to recover
any aortic flow.

Anionic and Cationic Modifications

    Tissue ischemia induces an unfavourable redistribution of
ions and therefore the potential protective effect of the
modification of anionic and cationic balance was investigated.

    Hearts were subjected to a two minute pre-ischemic period of
coronary infusion with a variety of solutions containing elevated
concentrations of one or more of the following:- potassium chloride,
potassium citrate, potassium aspartate and magnesium chloride.

The infusion of potassium chloride (16mmol) in the coronary tree prior to the ischemic period rapidly induced cardiac arrest and improved post-ischemic recovery so that hearts (n=6) subjected to 30 minutes ischemia recovered to 29.9 $\pm$ 8.0% of their control aortic flow rate. In additional experiments (n=6 for each group) 16mmol potassium chloride was replaced by 16mmol potassium aspartate or 16mmol potassium citrate. The recoveries were 28$\pm$ 7.6% and 11.1 $\pm$ 5.4% respectively. In a further series of experiments (n=6 for each group) hearts were subjected to pre-ischemic perfusion with solutions containing 16mmol potassium chloride plus 16mmol magnesium chloride or 16mmol potassium chloride plus 16mmol magnesium aspartate. The hearts were subjected to 30 minutes ischemia and after 15 minutes of the recovery period the hearts had recovered to 68.1 $\pm$ 5.7% and 73.6 $\pm$ 5.1% of the control aortic flow rate.

These combined results illustrate the marked protective action of potassium and also magnesium and show that their effects are additive. The striking protective action of both potassium and magnesium is possibly based on their ability to reverse unfavourable cellular ion losses and also their ability to induce cardiac arrest rapidly and so conserve the limited supplies of energy available during ischemia for cellular maintenance and protection. Contrary to the suggestions of Bretschneider (19) and Kirsch (21), the inclusion of aspartate does not significantly improve protection and recovery. The inclusion of citrate, which may have a potential damaging effect through its ability to chelate calcium or inhibit anaerobic glycolysis, significantly reduced the protection afforded by potassium.

Modification of Electrical Activity

Procaine has been suggested as an effective cardioplegic agent (21) and possibly may also act as a protective agent through its rapid induction of arrest and the prevention of ischemic beating. The ability of residual procaine to combat any rhythmic disturbance during recovery may add to its potential value. Hearts (n=6) were therefore infused, prior to ischemia, with perfusion fluid containing 7.4mmol procaine and this improved the recovery of aortic flow from 0 to 26.2 $\pm$ 19.4%.

Modification of Metabolic Activity

It is often suggested that glucose in combination with potassium and insulin may be able to protect the ischemic or hypoxic myocardium (25,26,27,28,29). Studies were therefore carried out to determine whether the inclusion of glucose and insulin in an infusate was able to improve the recovery of the

TABLE I

The effect of glucose and insulin upon the recovery of aortic
flow in hearts subjected to 30 minutes of normothermic ischemia.
The concentrations of the agents in the pre-ischemic infusates
were potassium, 16mmol; Magnesium 16mmol; Glucose 11mmol; Insulin
0.01 iu/ml.

INFUSATE COMPOSITION	% RECOVERY OF AORTIC FLOW
BUFFER + HIGH K^+ + HIGH Mg^{++}	$68.1 \pm 5.7\%$
BUFFER + HIGH K^+ + HIGH Mg^{++} + GLUCOSE	$66.5 \pm 8.1\%$
BUFFER + HIGH K^+ + HIGH Mg^{++} + GLUCOSE + INSULIN	$65.8 \pm 3.1\%$

TABLE II

The additive and protective effects of potassium (16mmol),
Magnesium (16mmol), Adenosine Triphosphate (10mmol), Creatine
Phosphate (10mmol) and Procaine (7.4mmol) in the pre-ischemic
infusate upon the recovery of aortic flow rate after 30 minutes
of normothermic ischemia.

INFUSATE COMPOSITION	% RECOVERY OF AORTIC FLOW
BUFFER	%
BUFFER + HIGH K^+	$29.9 \pm 8.0\%$
BUFFER + HIGH K^+ + HIGH Mg^{++}	$68.1 \pm 5.7\%$
BUFFER + HIGH K^+ + ATP	$76.6 \pm 4.4\%$
BUFFER + HIGH K^+ + CP + PROCAINE	$63.5 \pm 12.7\%$
BUFFER + HIGH K^+ + ATP + HIGH Mg^{++}	$86.8 - 0.9\%$
BUFFER + HIGH K^+ + ATP + HIGH Mg^{++} + CP + PROCAINE	$93.1 \pm 1.0\%$

ischemic and the ischemic arrested heart. Hearts (n=6 for each
group) were infused with perfusion fluid containing 16mmol potassium
plus 16mmol magnesium with and without 11mmol glucose and/or 0.01iu/ml
insulin. The results revealed that the inclusion of glucose or
insulin did not improve post-ischemic recovery (Table 1).

Extracellular high energy phosphates have also been suggested
(30,31,32) as potential protective agents. Hearts (n=6 for each
group) were therefore perfused with various combinations of
protective agents including 10mmol adenosine triphosphate and 10mmol
creatine phosphate. The results (Table 2) in addition to revealing
the striking protective action of extracellular adenosine triphosphate
and creatine phosphate also revealed that the protective effects of
potassium, magnesium, procaine, adenosine triphosphate and creatine
phosphate are additive.

Modification of the Temperature of the Ischemic Myocardium

The well known protective effects of hypothermia (1,2,16,17,18,
19) was investigated in relation to the protective agents studied
above. Hearts (n=6 for each group) were infused with buffer
containing 12mmol potassium plus 16mmol adenosine triphosphate
plus 1.0mmol procaine. The hearts were then subjected to 60 minutes
of ischemia at increasing temperatures. At the end of the recovery
period the hearts had recovered to $95.8 \pm 1.2\%$ at $4°C$, $92.4 \pm 2.5\%$
at $12°C$, $86.7 \pm 3.9\%$ at $20°C$, $83.8 \pm 2.4\%$ at $25°C$, $75.1 \pm 1.0\%$ at
$28°C$, $57.5 \pm 7.1\%$ at $30°C$, $9.7 \pm 5.0\%$ at $33°C$ and 0% at $37°C$.

DISCUSSION

The work reported in this paper has evaluated, individually and
in combination, a variety of potentially protective interventions
with a view to devising an effective means of myocardial protection.
The results of the studies stress the potential of this approach
as hearts which would normally fail totally to recover after 30
minutes of ischemia can be made to recover to almost 100% of their
pre-ischemic function after 60 minutes of ischemia, simply by the
use of an appropriate intervention. Figure 3 illustrates how
post-ischemic recovery can be progressively improved with the use
of these interventions.

Our studies have involved the infusion of various aqueous
solutions into the coronary tree just prior to the onset of
ischemia. Our results suggest that effective protection can
be resolved into two distinct components: the rapid induction
of cardiac arrest and the ability of some compounds to combat
specific deleterious changes in the muscle.

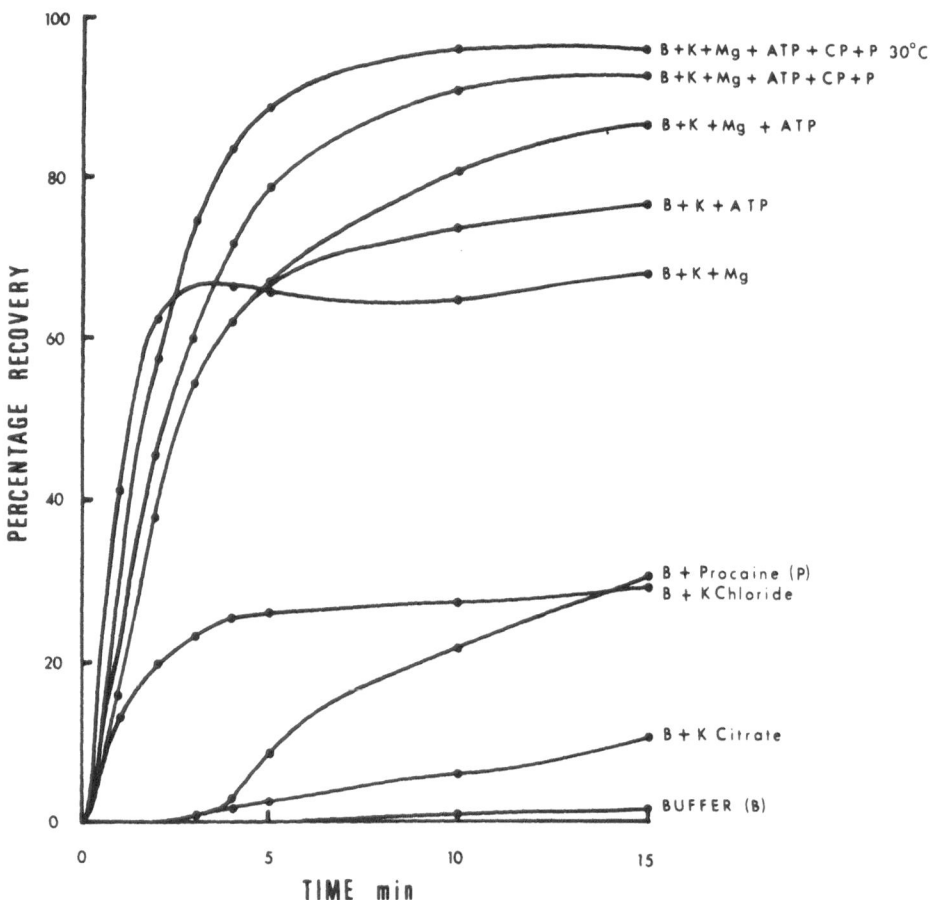

Figure 3
The efficacy of various pre-ischemic infusates for the improvement
of post-ischemic recovery of aortic flow in the isolated rat
heart after a 30 minute period of bypass.

Immediately following the onset of myocardial ischemia there is a reduction of contractile activity, but some contraction continues for several minutes and may recur later. Cardioplegic agents such as potassium or procaine induce instantaneous cardiac arrest and thereby conserve vital cellular energy supplies for the maintenance of morphological and biochemical integrity and subsequent recovery.

The second component relies on the ability, in theory at least, of certain compounds to combat one or more of the deleterious changes which occur as a result of tissue ischemia. Potassium and magnesium may exert their protective effect by reducing intracellular ion losses. Procaine, like potassium, in addition to inducing rapid cardiac arrest, may exert an additional protective action by reducing the incidence of dysrhythmias during the recovery period. The effects of intracellular adenosine triphosphate and creatine phosphate are of particular interest. It is commonly held that cell membranes are impermeable to high energy phosphates but there have been several reports in the literature (30,33) suggesting that adenosine triphosphate is in fact able to cross the muscle cell membrane. Whether the extracellular high energy phosphates enter the cell or whether they act on the cell membrane is unknown, but their protective effect is striking and is additive to that of potassium, magnesium and procaine.

Topical hypothermia for the duration of ischemia, through its ability to reduce metabolic rate, energy consumption and degradative processes, can be a powerful adjunct to the protective action of various infusates. The greater the degree of hypothermia the greater the protection in these results.

In conclusion, these findings, though limited by their observation in the rat heart, emphasise the striking value of pre-ischemic infusions in counteracting the deleterious cellular changes induced by myocardial ischemia. The use of carefully formulated infusates in the human heart before periods of ischemia, such as aortic occlusion during open heart surgery, may permit a considerable extension of the duration of ischemia that can be tolerated by the heart with complete functional recovery.

REFERENCES

1. Hearse, D.J., Stewart, D.A., Chain, E.B.: Recovery from
    cardiac bypass and elective cardiac arrest: Metabolic
    consequences of various cardioplegic procedures in the
    isolated rat heart. Circ.Res. 35: 448-457,1974.

2. Hearse, D.J., Stewart, D.A., Braimbridge, M.B.: Hypothermic
    arrest and potassium arrest: Metabolic and myocardial
    protection during elective cardiac arrest. Circ.Res.36:
    481-489,1975.

3. Melrose, D.G., Dreyer, B., Bentall, H.H., Baker, J.B.E.:
    Elective cardiac arrest. Lancet 2: 21-22,1955.

4. Bernhard, W.F., Schwartz, H.F., Mallick, N.P.: Elective
    hypothermic cardiac arrest in normothermic animals. Ann.
    Surg. 153: 43-51,1961.

5. Sealy, W.C., Young, W.G., Brown, I.W., Harris, J.S.,
    Merritt, D.H.: Potassium, magnesium and neostigmine for
    controlled cardioplegia. J.Thorac.Cardiovasc.Surg.37:655-659,
    1959.

6. Hurley, E.J., Lower, R.R., Dong, E., Pillsbury, R.C.,
    Shumway, N.E.: Clinical experience with local hypothermia
    in elective cardiac arrest. J.Thorac.Cardiovasc.Surg.
    47: 50-65,1964.

7. Bloodwell, R.D., Kidd, J.N., Hallman, G.L., Burdette, W.J.,
    McMurtrey, M.J., Cooley, D.A.: Cardiac valve replacement
    without coronary perfusion: Clinical and laboratory
    observations. In Prosthetic Heart Valves edited by L.A.
    Brewer. Springfield, Illinois, Charles C. Thomas, pp 397-410,
    1969.

8. Cooley, D.A., Reul, G.J., Wukasch, D.C.: Ischemic contracture
    of the heart: "Stone Heart" Am.J.Cardiol. 29:575-577,1972.

9. Greenberg, J.J., Edmunds, L.H., Brown, R.B.: Myocardial
    metabolism and post-arrest function in the cold and
    chemically arrested heart. Surgery 48:31-42,1960.

10. Tyres, G.F.O., Todd, G.J., Neeley, J.R., Waldhausen, J.A.:
    The mechanism of myocardial protection from ischemic arrest
    by intracoronary tetrodotoxin administration. J.Thorac.
    Cardiovasc.Surg. 69:190-195,1975.

11. Iyengar, S.R.K., Ramchand,S., Charrette, E.J.P., Iyengar,
    C.K.S., Lynn, R.B.: Anoxic cardiac arrest: Experimental

and clinical study of its effects. J.Thorac.Cardiovasc.
Surg. 66:722-730,1973.

12. Braimbridge, M.V., Darracott, S., Clement, A.J., Bitensky,
     L., Chayen, J.: Myocardial deterioration during aortic
     valve replacement assessed by cellular biological tests.
     J.Thorac.Cardiovasc.Surg. 66:241-246,1973.

13. Reis, R.L., Staroscik, R.N., Rodgers, B.M., Enright, L.P.,
     Morrow, A.G.: Left ventricular function after ischemic
     cardioplegia. Arch.Surg. 99:815-820,1969.

14. Jennings, R.B., Sommers, H.M., Hudson, P.B., Kretenbach,
     J.P.: Ischemic injury of myocardium. Ann. N.Y. Acad.Sci.
     156: 61-78, 1969.

15. Gott, V.L., Bartlett, M., Johnson, J.A., Long, D.M.,
     Lillehei, C.W.: High energy phosphate levels in the human
     heart during potassium citrate arrest and selective
     hypothermic arrest. Surg. Forum 10; 544-547, 1960.

16. Griepp, R.B., Stinson, E.B., Shumway, N.E.: Profound
     local hypothermia for myocardial protection during open
     heart surgery. J.Thorac.Cardiovasc.Surg. 66:731-739,1973.

17. Proctor, E.: Early sinus rhythm in dog hearts preserved
     for 96 hours and assessed ex vivo. Transplantation 13:
     437-438, 1972.

18. Levy, M.N.,: Oxygen consumption and blood flow in the
     hypothermic, perfused kidney. Am.J.Physiol. 197:1111-1114,
     1959.

19. Bretschneider, H.J.: Uberlebenszeit und Wiederbelebungszeit
     des Herzens bei Normo-und Hypothermie. Verh Dtsch Ges
     Kreislaufforsch 30: 11-34, 1964.

20. Kirsch, U., Rodewald, G., Kalmar, P.: Induced ischemic
     arrest. J.Thorac.Cardiovasc.Surg 63: 121-130, 1972.

21. Kirsch, U.: Untersuchungen zum Eintritt der Totenstarre
     an ischaemischen Meerschweinchenherzen in Normothermie.
     Der Winfluss von Procaine, Kalium un Magnesium, Arzneim.
     Forsch 20; 1071-1074, 1970.

22. Neely, J.R., Liebermeister, H., Battersby, E.J., Morgan, H.E.:
     Effect of pressure development on oxygen consumption by
     isolated rat heart. Am.J. Physiol. 212: 804-814, 1967.

23. Langendorff, O.: Untersuchungen am überlebenden Säugethier-
    herzen. Pfluegers Arch. 61: 291-332, 1958.

24. Krebs, H.A., Henseleit, K.: Untersuchungen über die Harnstoff-
    bildung im Tierkörper. Hoppe Seylers Z. Physiol. Chem. 210:
    33-66, 1932.

25. Weissler, A.M., Kruger, G.A., Baba, N., Scarpelli, D.G.,
    Leighton, R.D., Gallimore, J.K.: The role of anaerobic
    metabolism in the preservation of functional capacity and
    structure of anoxic myocardium. J.Clin.Invest. 47:403-416,
    1968.

26. Opie, L.H.: The glucose hypothesis: relation to acute
    myocardial ischemia. J.Molec.Cell.Cardiol. 1: 107-115, 1970.

27. Brachfeld, W.: Ischemic myocardial metabolism and cell necrosis.
    Bull N.Y. Acad.Med. 50: 261-293, 1974.

28. Hearse, D.J., Chain, E.B.: The role of glucose in the survival
    and recovery of the anoxic isolated perfused rat heart.
    Biochem. J. 128:1125-1133, 1972.

29. Hearse, D.J., Humphrey, S.M.: Enzyme release during myocardial
    anoxia: a study of metabolic protection. J.Molec.Cell
    Cardiol. 7: 463-482, 1975.

30. Wilkinson, J.H., Robinson, J.M.: Effects of energy rich
    compounds on release of intracellular enzymes from human
    leukocytes and rat lymphocytes. Clin.Chem. 20: 1331-1336,
    1974.

31. Parratt, J.R., Marshall, R.J.: The response of isolated
    cardiac muscle to acute anoxia: protective effect of adenosine
    triphosphate and creatine phosphate. J.Pharm.Pharmac.
    26: 427-433, 1974.

32. Fedelesova, M., Ziegelhoffer, A., Krause, E.G., Wollenberger,
    A.: Effect of exogenous adenosine triphosphate upon the
    metabolic state of the excised hypothermic dog heart.
    Cir.Res. XXIV: 617-727, 1969.

33. Chaudry, I.H., Gould, M.K.: Evidence for the uptake of ATP
    by rat soleus muscle in vitro. Biochem. Biophys. Acta
    196: 320-326, 1970.

Part III

RECONSTRUCTION OF THE RIGHT VENTRICULAR OUTFLOW TRACT

THE OUTFLOW TRACT AND PULMONARY ARTERIES IN FALLOT'S TETRALOGY AND PULMONARY ATRESIA WITH VENTRICULAR SEPTAL DEFECT

T. A. H. ENGLISH

REGIONAL CARDIOTHORACIC UNIT

PAPWORTH HOSPITAL, CAMBRIDGE, CB3 8RE

The subject of this symposium is the surgical reconstruction of the right ventricular outflow tract. This presentation describes relevant aspects of the pathological anatomy encountered in Fallot's tetralogy and pulmonary atresia with ventricular septal defect. Time does not permit consideration of the abnormal outflow tract in double outlet right ventricle and transposition complexes.

As with most operations for congenital heart disease, successful surgical treatment depends upon the accurate delineation of abnormal anatomy pre-operatively, so that the appropriate repair can be logically planned. Knowledge of the normal anatomy and a method of categorizing variations from the normal are both necessary. Failure to obtain general acceptance of an agreed terminology to describe structures in the right ventricular outflow tract has been responsible for much confusion and a clear definition of anatomical terms is therefore necessary.

DEFINITION OF TERMS AND NORMAL ANATOMY

The normal right ventricle has an inflow portion (sinus or body) and an outflow portion or infundibulum. The embryological term "conus" has been used synonymously with the anatomical term "infundibulum" and this has been the source of considerable misunderstanding. In 1966, Van Praagh defined the conus as constituting the muscular segment between the semilunar and atrioventricular valves. Recognizing that this failed to delineate the inferior limit of its free wall in the normally developed heart, Goor and Edwards (1970) proposed that the conus

be defined as that part of the right ventricle which lies between
the pulmonary valve above, and an imaginary line through the
papillary muscle of the conus and the upper edge of the membranous
septum below. However, on examination of the normal right ventricle, inflow and outflow portions appear clearly demarcated by a
muscular annulus formed by parietal and septal trabeculae extending
from the lower part of the infundibular septum to meet on the free
wall of the right ventricle just above the insertion of the
moderator band. We would therefore define the right ventricular
infundibulum as lying between this plane below and the pulmonary
valve above (Fig. 1).

The infundibular septum, which separates the right and left
pulmonary cusps from the tricuspid valve, is shorter than the
infundibular free wall and is comprised of several distinct
anatomical structures (Fig. 2). Centrally, the conal septum
(embryologic conus) separates the aortic and pulmonary outflow
tracts and is continuous laterally with the parietal trabeculum
("parietal band"). Deep to the parietal part of the conal septum
is the conoventricular flange. This is a small segment of
ventricular musculature that remains unabsorbed between atrial and
bulbar segments of the primitive heart tube after the looping

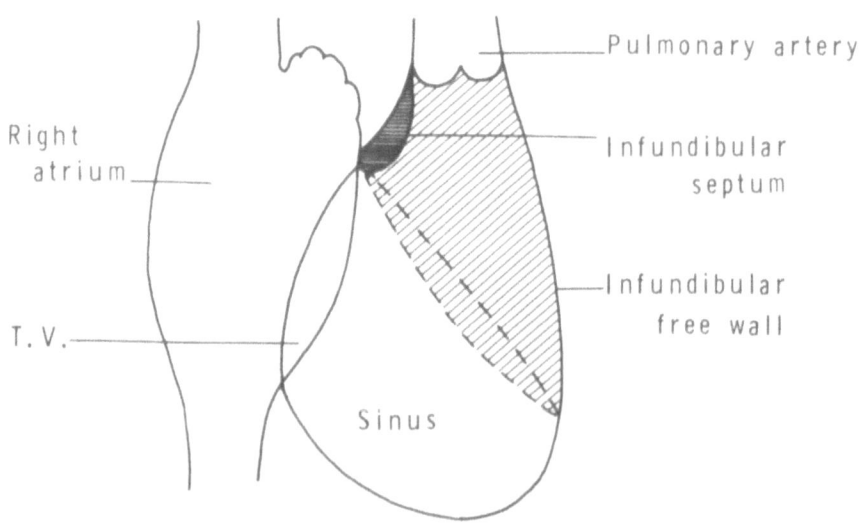

Right Ventricle

Inflow portion (sinus) +

Outflow portion (infundibulum)

Figure 1

Normal

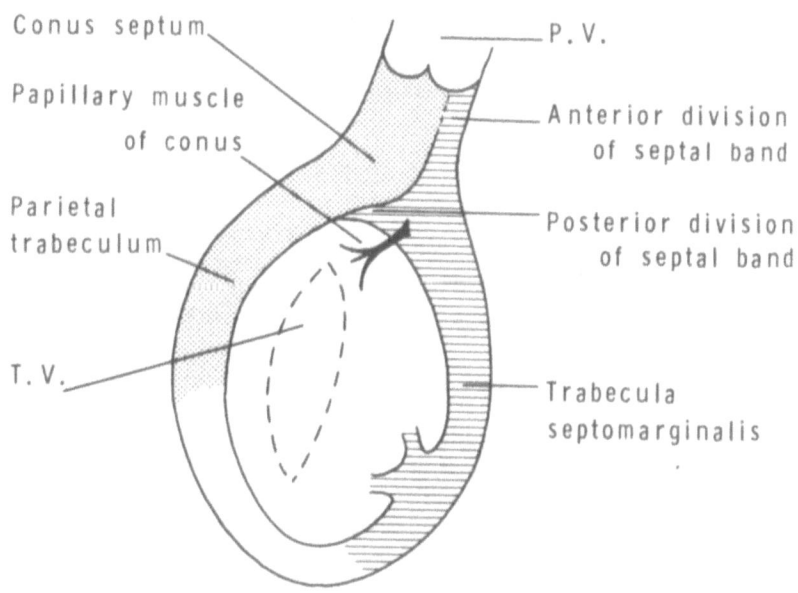

Conus septum

Papillary muscle
    of conus

Parietal
trabeculum

T.V.

P.V.

Anterior division
    of septal band

Posterior division
    of septal band

Trabecula
septomarginalis

Figure 2

process has taken place. During normal development of the heart,
the middle part of the conoventricular flange is absorbed as
the aortic outflow comes in contact with the left ventricle
(Anderson et al, 1974). The right extension of the flange persists
to separate the aortic valve from the tricuspid valve. Medially,
the conal septum is in conjunction with the anterior and posterior
divisions of the septal component of the trabecula septomarginalis
(Fig. 2). The latter is a broad mass of muscle on the septal
surface of the right ventricle comprising both septal and moderator
bands. At its superior extent, the septal band divides into an
anterior limb, which passes up towards the pulmonary valve, and
a posterior limb from which arises the papillary muscle of the
conus. Inferiorly, the moderator band crosses the right ventricular cavity to fuse with the parietal extension of the conal
septum. The anterior papillary muscle of the tricuspid valve
arises from the trabecula septomarginalis towards the ventricular
apex. The trabecula septomarginalis is derived embryologically
from the proximal bulbus (primitive right ventricular sinus) and
is seldom involved in what are ordinarily regarded as conotruncal
malformations (an exception is that condition known as anomalous
muscle bundle of the right ventricle, which probably represents

high and obstructive septal and moderator bands). Indeed,
Van Praagh (1973) has stressed that "only by happy normalcy do
the parietal and septal bands come together to form the structure
known as the crista supraventricularis". We agree with Becker
and colleagues (1975) that until a standard nomenclature has been
adopted, the term crista supraventricularis is preferably restric-
ted to the right ventricular structure seen in normal hearts.

THE OUTFLOW TRACT IN FALLOT'S TETRALOGY

Obstruction to flow from the right ventricle in Fallot's
tetralogy is due to varying degrees of narrowing of the infundibulum, the pulmonary annulus and valve, the main pulmonary trunk,
and the right and left pulmonary arteries.

The morphogenesis of the infundibular obstruction remains
controversial. Van Praagh (1970) has suggested that the primary
aetiological event is underdevelopment of the subpulmonary conus
and that all other anatomical characteristics, such as the anterior
position of the ventricular septal defect, the overriding of the
aorta, and the relative posterior, inferior and leftward displace-
ment of the pulmonary valve are secondary to this. This view has
been challenged by Goor and colleagues (1971) and by Becker and
colleagues (1975) who conclude that Fallot's tetralogy results
from a combination of conotruncal malrotation and malseptation.
The former causes dextroposition of the aorta, whereas the latter
gives rise to "hypoplasia" of the infundibulum (Fig. 3). This
results from anterior deviation of the conal septum, which is
manifest morphologically by separation of its parietal insertion
from the conoventricular flange. This usually continues to
persist between aorta and tricuspid valves but may become further
absorbed giving rise to an area of aortic-tricuspid continuity.
The ventricular septal defect is due to failure of the conal
septum to fill the space above the posterior division of the
septal band and the ventricular septum (Fig. 4).

Whatever the precise embryogenesis of the infundibular
narrowing, secondary hypertrophy of the muscular components
forming the annulus between sinus and infundibulum of right
ventricle may contribute significantly to the obstruction to
outflow. Hypertrophy of the parietal extension of the conal
septum and the anterior division of the septal band is particularly
important and may result in the angiographic appearance of fore-
shortening of the infundibulum. However, the elegant morphometric
studies of Becker and colleagues (1975) have shown that infundibular length, expressed as a ratio of the length of the infundibular
septum to the length of the right ventricle from apex to pulmonary
valve, is no shorter in Fallot's tetralogy than in the normal
heart.

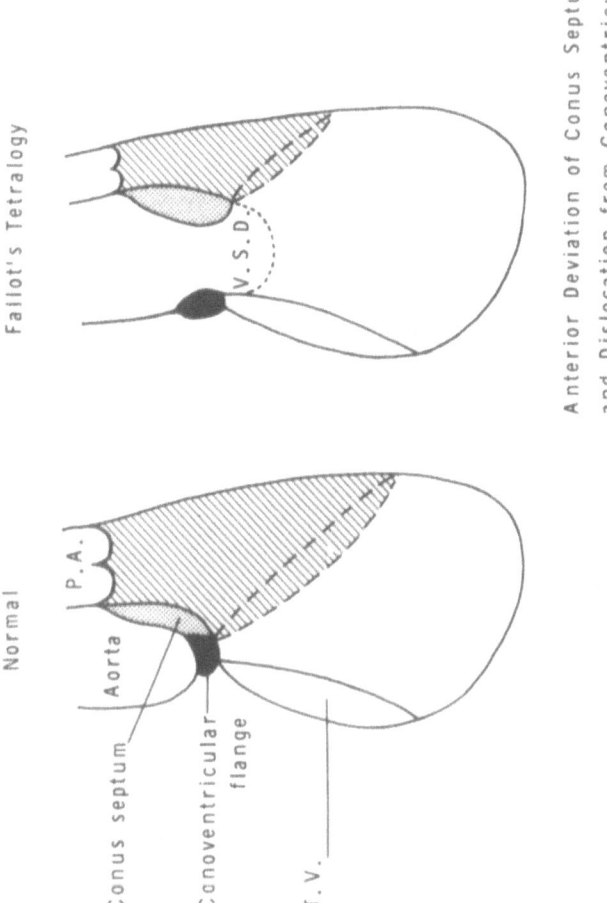

Figure 3

Fallot's Tetralogy

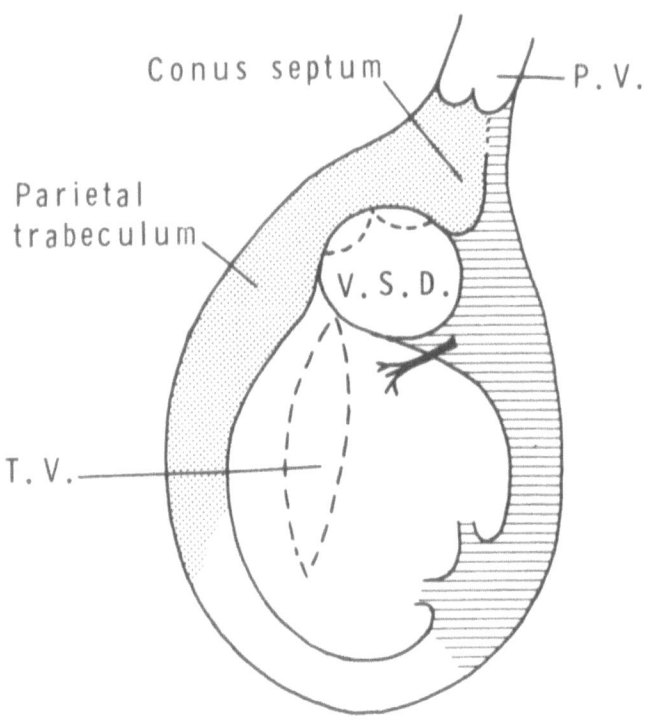

Figure 4

The nature of the outflow tract obstruction may be one factor
in determining the site of ventriculotomy and despite wide individual variations in morphology, attempts have been made to
classify the sites of obstruction (Brock, 1957; Hawe et al, 1970;
Utley & Roe, 1973). Of these, the classification presented by
the Mayo Clinic group is one of the most satisfactory and is
illustrated in Fig. 5.

THE PULMONARY VALVE AND PULMONARY ARTERIES IN FALLOT'S TETRALOGY

Malformations affecting the pulmonary valve and annulus, the
pulmonary trunk, and the pulmonary arteries in Fallot's tetralogy
are listed in Table I.

Site of Outflow Tract Obstruction in Fallot's Tetralogy
(After McGoon (1970) - 202 Patients)

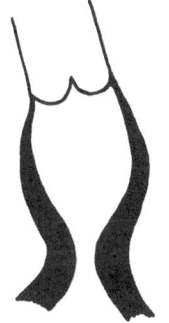 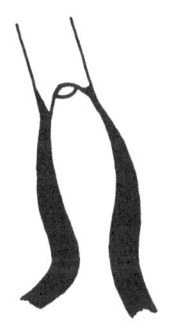 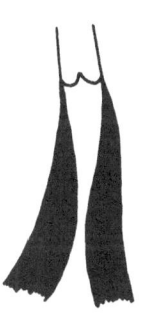 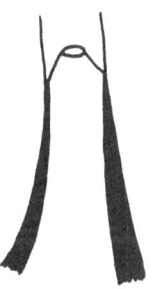

Isolated Infundibular (39%)	Infundibular and Valvar (35%)	Diffuse Hypoplasia (25%)	Isolated Valvar (1%)

Figure 5

TABLE I

ABNORMALITIES OF

PULMONARY VALVE AND ARTERIES IN FALLOT'S TETRALOGY

1. Hypoplasia of Pulmonary Annulus and Valve

2. Hypoplasia of Pulmonary Trunk and Pulmonary Arteries

3. Discrete Stenosis of Pulmonary Trunk

4. Peripheral Pulmonary Artery Stenosis

5. Absent Pulmonary Valve

6. Absent Left Pulmonary Artery

7. Origin of Pulmonary Artery from Aorta

Pure infundibular obstruction, no matter how severe, can
usually be relieved by adequate resection of muscle. When reconstruction with an outflow patch is necessary, this is generally
because of the presence of a small pulmonary annulus, or the
association of a small pulmonary annulus with hypoplasia of the
pulmonary trunk, which may extend peripherally into the origin
of the left or right pulmonary arteries (Fig. 6). Very occasionally, a localised stricture of the pulmonary trunk is encountered
and an example of this is illustrated in Figure 7. At operation
the presence of a ring stenosis 6 mm. in diameter and situated
just proximal to the bifurcation of the pulmonary trunk was
confirmed. This was treated by a separate pericardial patch
angioplasty, in addition to the usual infundibular resection and
closure of ventricular septal defect. Peripheral pulmonary
arterial stenoses are rare in Fallot's tetralogy but may occasionally be the source of a continuous murmur (Ongley et al, 1966).

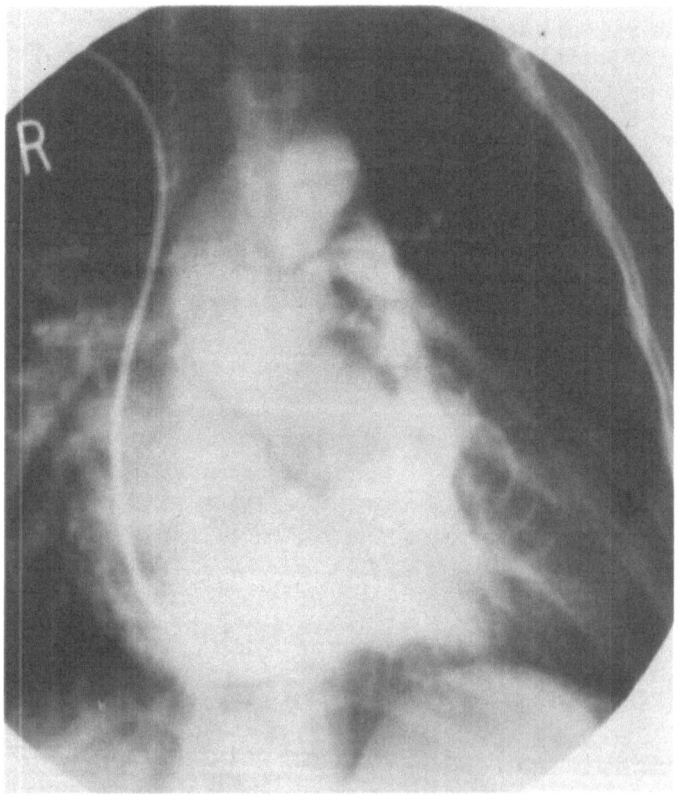

Fig. 6. Right ventricular angiocardiogram in a patient with hypoplasia of the pulmonary annulus, pulmonary trunk, and origin of
left pulmonary artery.

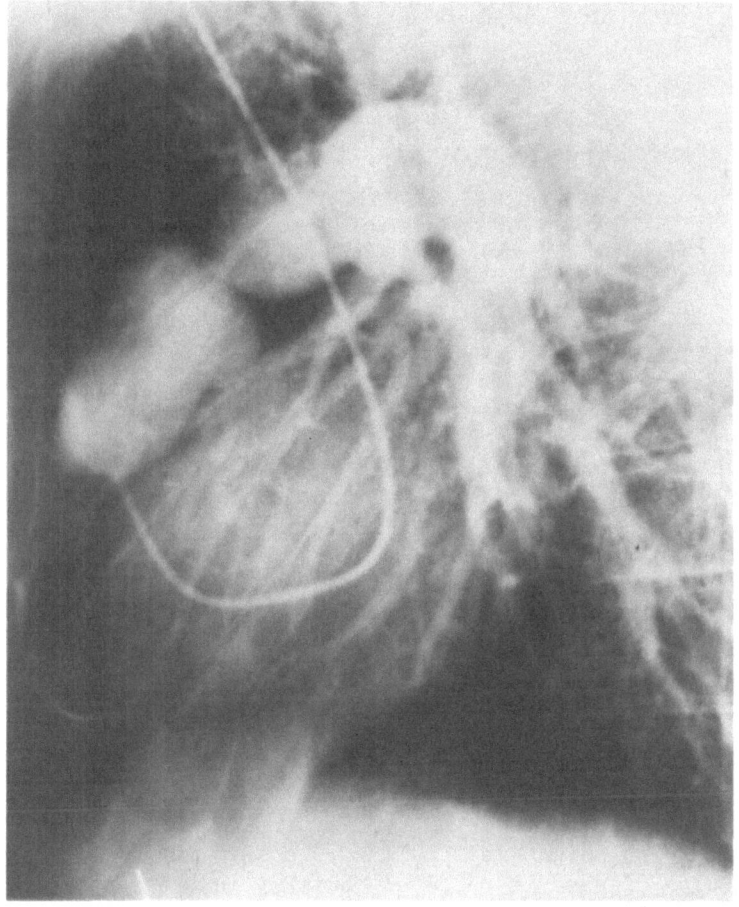

Fig. 7. Lateral angiocardiogram. Injection into infundibulum
showing a ring stenosis of the pulmonary trunk.

The syndrome of absent pulmonary cusps with aneurysmal
dilatation of the pulmonary trunk and proximal pulmonary arteries
occurs in about 3% of surgical cases of tetralogy of Fallot
(Stafford et al, 1973). The pulmonary annulus is usually narrowed,
resulting in pressure gradients both at this site and at infundibular level. Extreme dilatation of the pulmonary arteries may
compress adjoining structures and give rise to respiratory obstruction in infancy. Figure 8 is the right ventriocular angiogram of
a patient with absent pulmonary valve and also congenital absence
of the left pulmonary artery. Successful reconstruction of the
outflow tract with an aortic valve homograft was accomplished and
we agree with Layton and colleagues (1972) that this is a more

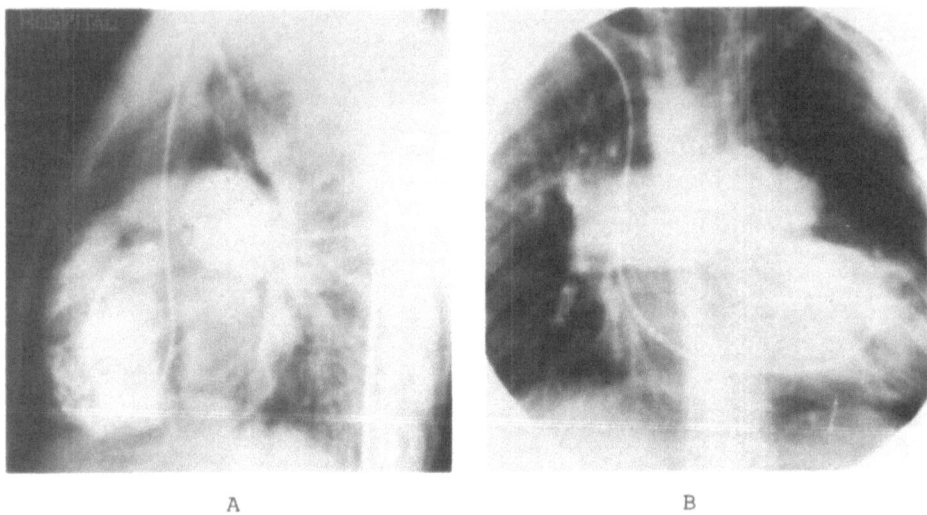

A   B

Fig. 8. A. Lateral projection in a patient with Fallot's tetralogy
and absent pulmonary valve. B. Anteroposterior projection in
same patient, showing congenital absence of left pulmonary artery.

satisfactory method of repair than simple relief of outflow tract
obstruction without the insertion of a valve (Stafford et al, 1973).

    Children with absent left pulmonary artery may develop pul-
monary vascular disease inordinately quickly in the right lung, so
that primary repair at an early age is desirable. Congenital
absence of the right pulmonary artery with Fallot's tetralogy has
yet to be recorded.

    Anomalous origin of either right or left pulmonary artery
from the ascending aorta in Fallot's tetralogy is very rare and
may not be diagnosed during pre-operative investigations. Routine
demonstration of the origin of both vessels from the pulmonary
trunk at operation is therefore advisable (Kuers & McGoon, 1973).

PULMONARY ATRESIA WITH VENTRICULAR SEPTAL DEFECT

    The intracardiac morphology of pulmonary atresia and large
ventricular septal defect is similar to that of tetralogy of
Fallot with severe infundibular hypoplasia but is distinguished
by absence of direct continuity between the right ventricle and
the pulmonary circulation. The latter is also a feature of
truncus arteriosus and classifications have recently been presented

embracing both conditions (Edwards & McGoon, 1973; Kirklin 1973).
However, despite the similarity in right ventricular morphology,
the clinical and haemodynamic characteristics of pulmonary
atresia and truncus arteriosus are so dissimilar that we believe
they should continue to be classified separately.

The term pseudotruncus arteriosus has been used by some
synonymously with pulmonary atresia and ventricular septal
(Bharati et al, 1975), and by others to describe a certain type
of pulmonary atresia characterised by confluence of the pulmonary
arteries (Pacifico et al, 1974). In view of the semantic confusion
associated with its use in the past, we agree with Somerville
(1970) and Wilkinson and Acerete (1973) that the term "pseudotruncus" is best avoided altogether.

The two most important anatomical considerations relating
to the surgical repair of pulmonary atresia with ventricular septal
defect are the degree of hypoplasia of the pulmonary arterial
system, from the infundibulum to the pulmonary hilum, and the
source of blood supply to the lungs (Table II). The former
influences the method used for restoring continuity between the
right ventricle and the pulmonary arterial system, whereas the
latter has important implications with respect to the route
of surgical access (McGoon et al, 1975).

TABLE II

PULMONARY ATRESIA WITH V.S.D.

May be classified according to -

1. Anatomy of Pulmonary Trunk and Right and Left Pulmonary Arteries.

   Varying degrees of development of Pulmonary part of Truncus

   Arteriosus and sixth aortic arch.

2. Source of Blood Supply to the Lungs.

   a. Ductus arteriosus

   b. Bronchial collaterals

   c. Surgically created shunts

   (d. Persistent fifth aortic arch)

The morphogenesis of pulmonary atresia is dependent primarily on unequal partitioning of the conotruncus at the expense of the subpulmonary infundibulum, pulmonary valve and pulmonary trunk, and on varying degrees of underdevelopment of the derivatives of the sixth arch, which form the right and left pulmonary arteries and the ductus arteriosus.

Surgically it is helpful to consider the whole spectrum of pulmonary atresia, from the infundibulum proximally to the hilar arteries peripherally. A classification based on this concept is offered in Table III, each of the five types being further categorized by the source of blood supply to the lungs. The angiographic demonstration of the latter, by aortography and selective catheterization of collateral vessels where necessary, is an essential part of the diagnostic assessment of these patients (Chesler et al, 1974; Macartney et al, 1974). Only in this way can the important distinction be made between those patients who have true pulmonary arteries (however hypoplastic), who are potentially operable, from those with complete agenesis of the pulmonary arterial system (truncus type IV), who are anatomically inoperable. In addition, McGoon and colleagues (1975) have convincingly shown that the outcome of an otherwise successful operation can be jeopardized by failure to recognize and ligate large collateral arteries at the time of corrective repair.

TABLE III

CLASSIFICATION OF PULMONARY ATRESIA WITH LARGE V.S.D.

1. Isolated Infundibular Atresia (Acquired)

2. Atresia of Pulmonary Valve and Proximal Trunk

3. Diffuse Atresia of Pulmonary Trunk with Confluent Right
   and Left Pulmonary Arteries. ("Pseudotruncus arteriosus")

        a. Patent ductus arteriosus

        b. Bronchial collaterals

4. Pulmonary Atresia with Non-Confluent Pulmonary Arteries

        a. Independent ductal origins

        b. Bronchial collaterals

        c. Mixed

5. Pulmonary Arterial (Sixth Arch) Agenesis. (Truncus Type IV")

TYPE I

Infundibular or valvar atresia may occur as an acquired
phenomenon secondary to the surgical creation of a palliative
aorto-pulmonary shunt (Frater et al, 1966) and therefore consti-
tues one of the factors that need consideration when palliation
rather than primary corrective repair is advocated. This phenomenon is illustrated in Figure 9, which shows the angiograms of
a patient 21 years after the establishment of a right Blalock
anastomosis in early childhood for proven Fallot's tetralogy. At
subsequent operation, the presence of complete infundibular
atresia was confirmed and repair was accomplished by reconstruction
of the outflow tract with an aortic homograft valve.

TYPE II

Patients with atresia limited to the pulmonary valve and
proximal pulmonary trunk may be treated surgically either by
reconstruction of the outflow tract with some form of valve, or
by the use of a large pericardial onlay patch. Some controversy
exists as to the relative merits of these two procedures; our

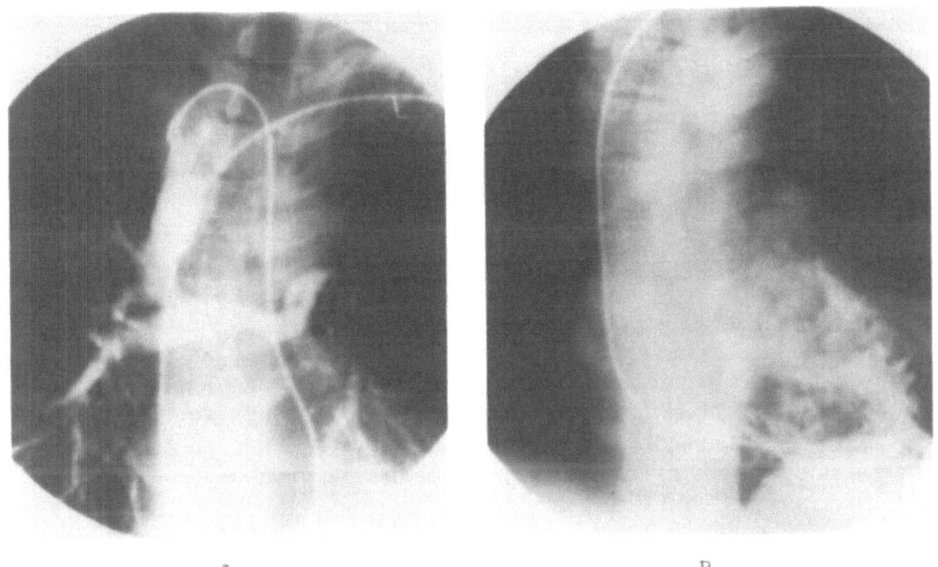

A   B

Fig. 9. A. Selective injection into right subclavian artery 21
years after Blalock-Taussig shunt for Fallot's tetralogy.
B. Right ventricular angiocardiogram in same patient showing
acquired infundibular atresia.

own belief is that the latter is satisfactory as a primary procedure for infants and young children in the absence of significant
pulmonary vascular disease, and in whom pulmonary incompetence
seems to be relatively well tolerated.

TYPE III

Where there is diffuse atresia of the whole pulmonary trunk,
some form of external valved conduit is necessary to restore continuity between the right ventricle and the confluence of the
right and left pulmonary arteries. In those cases presenting in
infancy, the blood supply to the lungs is often derived from a
persistent ductus arteriosus, whereas in older children it is
commoner to find that the pulmonary circulation is supplied from
large bronchial collateral arteries (McGoon et al, 1975). These
may be single or multiple and usually arise from the upper descending thoracic aorta or from the major arterial branches of the
aortic arch. They probably represent persistence and enlargement
of primitive intersegmental arteries originating from the dorsal
aorta and connecting with the vascular plexus of the primitive
lung bud before the development of the pulmonary arteries from
the sixth aortic arches (Jefferson et al, 1972). In contrast
with the diffuse small arterial collaterals found in Fallot's
tetralogy and other cyanotic conditions, which seem to develop
in response to cyanosis and progress with time, the persistence
of these vessels is probably related to failure of central pulmonary arterial development.

These large bronchial collateral arteries are tortuous,
thin-walled, and under systemic pressure. Stenoses at the junction
between them and the true pulmonary arteries afford a variable
degree of protection against the development of pulmonary vascular
disease. During operative repair, these vessels must be interrupted at the beginning of cardiopulmonary bypass and for this
purpose a technique of combined lateral thoracotomy and median
sternotomy was described by Doty and colleagues in 1972. We have
used a bilateral transverse submammary thoracotomy as an alternative
approach and have found that this gives excellent exposure, both
of the descending thoracic aorta and of the pulmonary vessels out
to the hilum. Figure 10 illustrates the angiograms of a patient
with Type III pulmonary atresia in whom this approach was used
successfully.

TYPE IV

Pulmonary atresia with hypoplastic or non-confluent right
and left pulmonary arteries may have pulmonary blood supply from
independent ductal origins, from large bronchial collateral

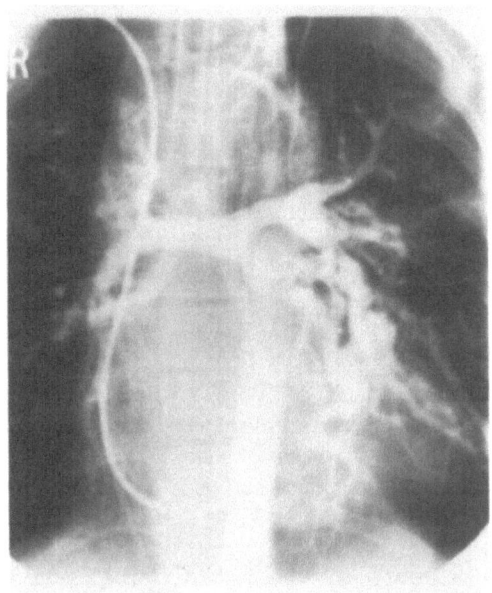

Fig. 10. Anteroposterior aortogram in a patient with Type III
Pulmonary atresia, with pulmonary blood supply from large
bronchial collateral vessels.

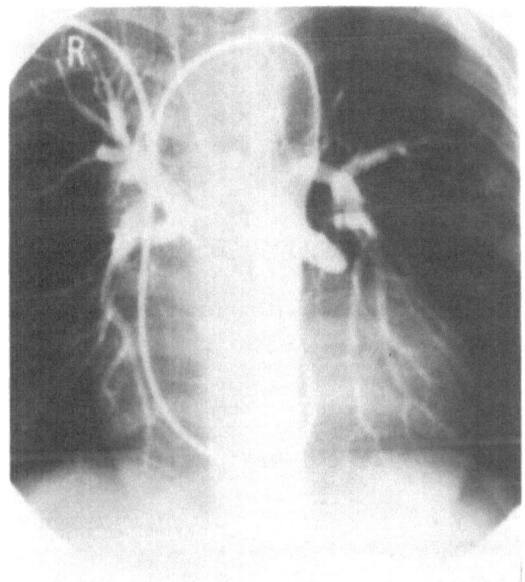

Fig. 11. Type IV Pulmonary atresia with non-confluent right and
left pulmonary arteries.

vessels, or from a mixture of both. Anatomically, it is most important to demonstrate the presence of true pulmonary arteries at the pulmonary hilum (Fig. 11) thereby distinguishing the condition from pulmonary arterial agenesis which is inoperable. Surgical repair necessitates the insertion of a bifurcating valved conduit after the ligation of all abnormal sources of blood supply to the lungs. The use of a bilateral transverse thoracotomy facilitates the construction of peripheral anastomoses at hilar level.

SUMMARY

Successful surgical repair of Fallot's tetralogy and pulmonary atresia with ventricular septal defect depends upon a knowledge of the normal anatomy and an appreciation of the varieties of outflow tract obstruction and pulmonary arterial malformations that may be encountered. Each case needs careful, individual assessment pre-operatively, with clear angiographic demonstration of all aspects of the pathological anatomy.

Two of the most important surgical considerations in pulmonary atresia with ventricular septal defect, are the degree of hypoplasia of the pulmonary arterial system and the source and nature of abnormal blood supply to the lungs. A classification based on these considerations is offered and illustrative examples presented.

REFERENCES

Anderson R.H., Wilkinson J.L., Arnold R., Lubkiewicz K: Morophogenesis of bulboventricular malformations. 1: Consideration of embryogenesis in the normal heart. Brit.Heart J. 36: 242, 1974.

Becker A.E., Connor M., Anderson R.H.: Tetralogy of Fallot: A morphometric and geometric study. Am. J. Cardiol. 35: 402, 1975.

Bharati S., Paul M.H., Idriss F.S., Potkin R.T., Lev M.: The surgical anatomy of pulmonary atresia with ventricular septal defect: Pseudotruncus. J. Thorac. Cardiovasc. Surg. 69: 713, 1975.

Brock R.C.: The anatomy of congenital pulmonary stenosis. Cassel & Company, London p.60, 1957.

Chesler E., Matisson R., Beck W.: The assessment of the arterial supply to the lungs in pseuodotruncus arteriosus and truncus arteriosus Type IV in relation to surgical repair. Am. Heart J: 543, 1974.

Doty D.B., Kouchoukos N.T., Kirklin J.W., Barcia A., Bargeron L.M.:
Surgery for pseudotruncus arteriosus with pulmonary blood flow
originating from upper descending thoracic aorta. Circulation
45 & 46 (Suppl. 1) I-121, 1972.

Edwards J.E., McGoon D.C.: Absence of anatomic origin from heart
of pulmonary arterial supply. Circulation 47: 393, 1973.

Frater R.W., Rudoph A.M., Hoffman J.I.E.: Acquired pulmonary
atresia in tetralogy of Fallot with a functioning Blalock-Taussig
shunt. Thorax 21: 457, 1966.

Goor D.A., Edwards J.E., Lillehei C.W.: The development of the
interventricular septum of the heart: Correlative morphogenic
study. Chest 58: 453, 1970.

Goor D.A., Lillehei C.W., Edwards J.E.: Ventricular septal defects
and pulmonic stenosis with and without dextroposition: Anatomic
features and embryologic implications. Chest 60: 117, 1971.

Hawe A., Rastelli G.C., Ritter D.G., DuShane J.W., McGoon D.C.:
Management of the right ventricular outflow tract in severe
tetralogy of Fallot. J. Thorac. Cardiovasc. Surg. 6: 131, 1970.

Jefferson K., Rees S., Somerville J.: Systemic arterial supply
to the lungs in pulmonary atresia and its relation to pulmonary
artery development. Brit. Heart J. 34: 418, 1972.

Kirklin J.W.: Surgical classification of congenital heart disease.
In, Advances in Cardiovascular Surgery, edited by J.W. Kirklin,
Grune & Stratton, New York, p. 5, 1973.

Kuers P.F.W., McGoon D.C.: Tetralogy of Fallot with aortic origin
of the right pulmonary artery. J. Thorac. Cardiovasc. Surg. 65:
327, 1973.

Layton C.A., McDonald A., McDonald L., Towers M., Weaver J.,
Yacoub M.: The syndrome of absent pulmonary valve. Total
correction with aortic valvular homografts. J. Thorac. Cardiovasc.
Surg. 63: 800, 1972.

Macartney F.J., Scott O., Deverall P.B.: Haemodynamic and
anatomical characteristics of pulmonary blood supply in pulmonary
atresia with ventricular septal defect - including a case of
persistent fifth aortic arch. Brit. Heart J. 36: 1049, 1974.

McGoon D.C., Baird D.K., Davis G.D.: Surgical management of large
bronchial collateral arteries with pulmonary stenosis or atresia.
Circulation 52: 109, 1975.

Ongley P.A., Rahimtoola S.H., Kincaid O.W., Kirklin J.W.:
Continuous murmurs in tetralogy of Fallot and pulmonary atresia
with ventricular septal defect. Am. J. Cardiol. 18: 821, 1966.

Pacifico A.D., Kirklin J.W., Bargeron L.M., Soto B.: Surgical
treatment of common arterial trunk with pseudotruncus arteriosus.
Circulation 49 & 50 (Suppl. II) II-20, 1974.

Somerville J.: Management of pulmonary atresia. Brit. Heart J.
32: 641, 1970.

Stafford E.G., Mair D.D., McGoon D.C., Danielson G.K.: Tetralogy
of Fallot with absent pulmonary valve. Surgical considerations
and results. Circulation 47 & 48 (Suppl. III) III-24, 1973.

Utley J.R., Roe B.B.: Surgical considerations in obstruction of
the right ventricular outflow tract. J. Thorac. Cardiovasc. Surg.
65: 391, 1973.

Van Praagh R., Van Praagh S.:   Isolated ventricular inversion.
A consideration of the morphogenesis, definition and diagnosis of
nontransposed and transposed great arteries. Am.J. Cardiol. 17:
395, 1966.

Van Praagh R., Van Praagh S., Nebesar R.A., Muster A.J., Sinha S.N.,
Paul M.H.: Tetralogy of Fallot: Underdevelopment of the pulmonary
infundibulum and its sequelae. Am. J. Cardiol. 26: 25, 1970.

Van Praagh R.: Conotruncal malformations. In, Heart Disease
in Infancy: Diagnosis and Surgical Management, edited by
B.G. Barratt-Boyes, J.M. Neutze, E.A. Harris, Churchill
Livingstone, Edinburgh, p. 189, 1973.

Wilkinson J.L., Acerete F.: Terminological pitfalls in congenital
heart disease. Reappraisal of some confusing terms, with an
account of a simplified system of basic nomenclature. Brit.
Heart J. 35: 1166, 1973.

THE HAEMODYNAMICS OF THE ABNORMAL OUTFLOW TRACT

F. MACARTNEY

CONSULTANT PAEDIATRIC CARDIOLOGIST

KILLINGBECK HOSPITAL AND GENERAL INFIRMARY, LEEDS

I have been asked to speak on this subject of the haemodynamics of the abnormal right ventricular outflow tract. It may be stenotic, regurgitant, or atretic. If the obstruction cannot be relieved by excision alone, bypass it with a valved conduit. That is how simple the pioneering work of Mr. D. Ross and others (Ross and Somerville, 1966; McGoon, Rastelli and Ongley, 1968, McGoon, Rastelli and Wallace, 1970; Ionescu, Macartney and Wooler, 1972; Doty et al., 1972; Bowman, Hancock and Malm, 1973) has made the practical haemodynamics of the abnormal right ventricular outflow tract. But, as so often happens, clearing away one problem reveals others, more subtle and previously unsuspected. The most startling of these problems is one which, I suspect, anybody involved on any scale with the surgery of tetralogy of Fallot, with or without pulmonary atresia, has met and been baffled by: the patient who goes for surgery with a low or normal pulmonary artery pressure and comes back from the operating theatre (if he is lucky) with a pulmonary artery pressure approaching or exceeding systemic and a normal left atrial and pulmonary venous pressure (Somerville, et al., 1974).

There can be only one explanation for this phenomenon, which is that there is an excessive resistance to blood flow through the pulmonary blood vessels connected to the right ventricle by the surgeon. Now if in such a case pulmonary resistance has been calculated pre-operatively and found to be low or normal, the first suspect in the plot has to be the measurement of pulmonary resistance. But even when such obvious sources of error as pulmonary venous desaturation and pulmonary venous hypertension have been eliminated, there remains a problem in some patients.

I would like to suggest that one important source of error in pre-operative measurement of pulmonary resistance is the failure to recognise the presence of multifocal pulmonary blood supply.

The expression 'focus' (Fig. 1) (Macartney, Scott and Deverall, 1974) was coined by analogy with a lens, which causes parallel rays of light to be drawn together into a focus, from which the rays diverge again. In just such a way the right side of the normal heart focuses blood down into the main pulmonary artery, from which blood again diverges into the numerous peripheral pulmonary arteries. A focus is therefore defined as <u>any isolated vessel or complex of vessels, lying between the 'original source' of pulmonary blood supply and the resistance determining pulmonary arteries which provides effective pulmonary blood supply from an essentially common pressure head throughout the focus.</u>

In the normal heart (Fig. 1A) the right ventricle is the 'original source' of pulmonary blood supply and the main central pulmonary arteries form the focus. By contrast, when pulmonary blood supply does not originate directly from the heart, the aorta forms the 'original' source. What forms the focus or foci in this situation is very variable. In the second example shown (Fig. 1B), the left and right dorsal sixth aortic arches, corresponding more or less to the intrapericardial right and left pulmonary arteries, form a single focus. Note that this is the case despite the fact that there are two separate aorto-pulmonary anastomoses, a patent ductus arteriosus and a surgical aorta/right pulmonary artery shunt.

In the third example, (Fig. 1C), the two sixth aortic arches, supplied by a major aorta-pulmonary-collateral (MAPCA), form one focus, whereas a second focus is formed by an isolated MAPCA perfusing a segment of lung which is effectively independent from the remainder of the lung. Notice the fact that though the pulmonary arteries are confluent (Edwards and McGoon, 1973) there is multifocal pulmonary blood supply. The existence of isolated MAPCAs in the presence of confluent pulmonary arteries, originally demonstrated in life and confirmed at autopsy in one patient at the National Heart Hospital (Jefferson, Rees and Somerville, 1973) has now been independently confirmed in Leeds, Cape Town and New York (Macartney, et al., 1973; Chesler, Matisson and Beck, 1974; Levin, et al., 1974). Yet in a recent review of 262 patients from the Mayo Clinic with absence of anatomic origin from the heart of the pulmonary arterial supply, this quite common finding appears to have gone unnoticed. (Berry et al., 1974).

When the sixth aortic arches are absent, (Fig. 1D), the pulmonary arteries cannot be described either as confluent or non-confluent, but pulmonary supply is usually multifocal.

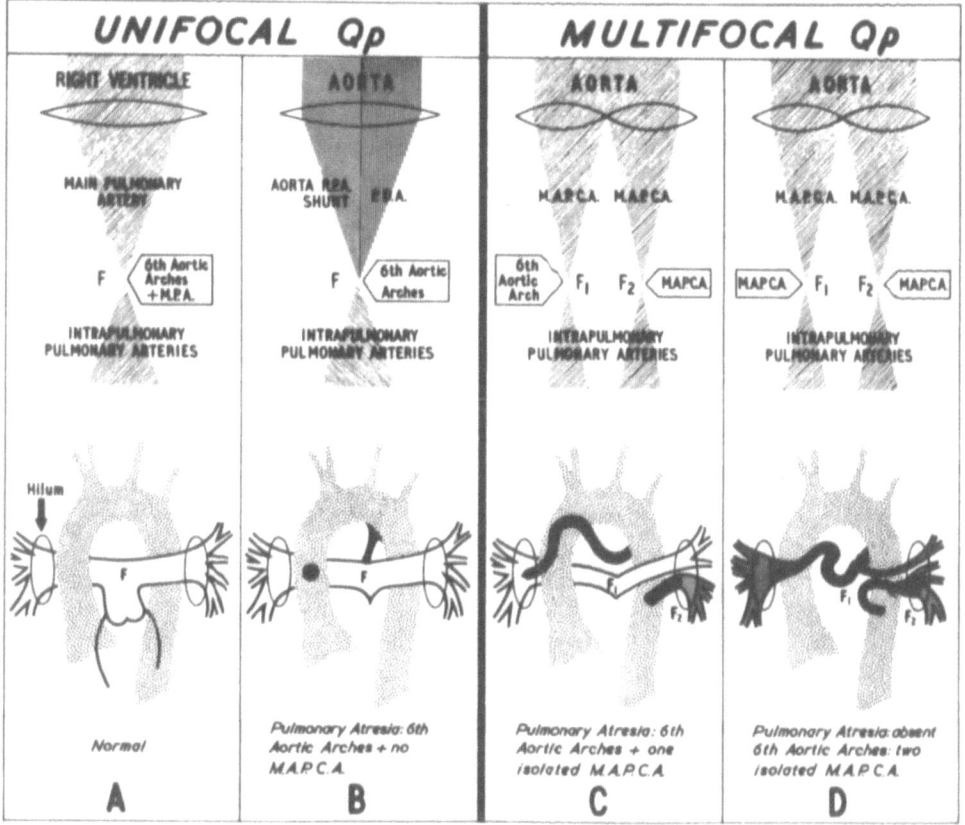

Figure 1

Diagrammatic illustration of unifocal and multifocal pulmonary blood supply (reproduced by kind permission of the British Heart Journal - (Macartney et al., 1974).

Reviewing the four varieties discussed, we can see that isolated MAPCAs indicate multifocal pulmonary supply. If however, for example, in Fig. 1B there is a stenosis of the right pulmonary blood supply without isolated MAPCAs and with confluent pulmonary arteries.

So, confluence and non-confluence of the pulmonary arteries are anatomical descriptions of the sixth aortic arch derivatives.

Unifocal and multifocal pulmonary blood supply are haemodynamic descriptions of the entire effective pulmonary blood supply. The only sense in which these two classifications correspond is that if the pulmonary arteries are non-confluent, then pulmonary blood supply must be multifocal.

What are the haemodynamic and surgical consequences of these
two major categories of pulmonary blood supply? By studying cases
of absence of the sixth aortic arch we were able to establish the
haemodynamic properties of MAPCAs (Macartney, Deverall and Scott,
1973). In brief, they are high resistance vessels. Much, if
not all, of this high resistance is the result of stenoses of the
arteries in the region of the hilum, where they anastamose with
the apparently normal intrapulmonary pulmonary arteries, which
are embryologic derivatives of the pulmonary plexuses. When
patients with pulmonary atresia with ventricular septal defect with
confluent pulmonary arteries were studied, these stenoses were
found to occur immediately before the MAPCA joined the sixth aortic
arches and pulmonary plexus derivatives, (Macartney et al., 1974).
These findings have been confirmed in patients investigated
subsequent to publication of those original reports.

Measurement of total pulmonary flow in pulmonary atresia is
relatively easy, since complete mixing of systemic and pulmonary
venous blood in the aortic root ensures that all blood entering
the pulmonary capillaries does so at the same oxygen saturation.
The Fick principle can therefore be applied with ease, provided
pulmonary venous saturation in the two lungs is equal, which it
normally is. However, if there is not pulmonary atresia, as for
example in straightforward tetralogy with a shunt, the blood
entering the pulmonary capillaries from the right ventricle will
have a lower oxygen saturation than the blood coming through the
shunt. This problem can be overcome by differential bronchospirometry, at least in older patients, (Fabricius and Rygg, 1971).

Measurement of total pulmonary resistance is relatively
straightforward when there is unifocal pulmonary blood supply. In
this case total pulmonary resistance is surgically relevant
information, since as a result of surgery the single focus will be
transferred from the aorta to the right ventricle.

If pulmonary blood supply is multifocal, total pulmonary
resistance can be determined with little error provided that the
mean pressures at the different foci are within 10mm/Hg of one-
another, and there is no gross maldistribution of blood as between
one focus and another, Macartney et al., 1973). However, the
answer obtained is only surgically relevant if at the end of
radical surgery all foci can be transferred from the aorta to the
right ventricle without any additional obstruction to pulmonary
blood flow being produced. Since this is usually not a practical
possibility, the surgically relevant question is what is the
pulmonary resistance relative to the focus or foci which can be
transferred to the right ventricle. There is at present no
completely satisfactory way of answering this question, since it
depends on the measurement of regional pulmonary flow and resistance.

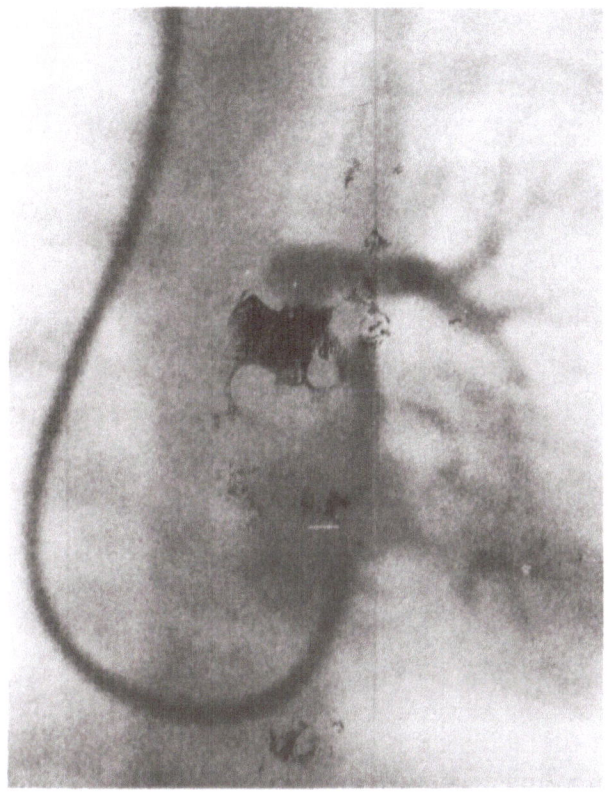

Figure 2

Fallot's tetralogy with multifocal pulmonary blood supply.
Frontal view of right ventricular angiocardiogram.

To illustrate the practical significance of this point, let
us suppose that in the patient represented in Fig. 1C, with
confluent pulmonary arteries and one isolated MAPCA, that only
10% of total pulmonary blood supply goes through the sixth aortic
arches and 90% through the isolated MAPCA. Let us suppose that
the mean sixth aortic arch pressure is normal and total pulmonary
flow is normal, i.e., equal to systemic. If we had failed to
observe the isolated MAPCA we might well conclude that following
radical surgery the mean pulmonary artery pressure would be
normal. In point of fact, however, if systemic output is maintained
and the MAPCA is ligated, there will be a blood flow through the
sixth aortic arches nine times greater post-operatively than
pre-operatively. We should not be surprised if the patient has
post-operative pulmonary hypertension.

So I hope you can follow the reasoning behind my suggestion

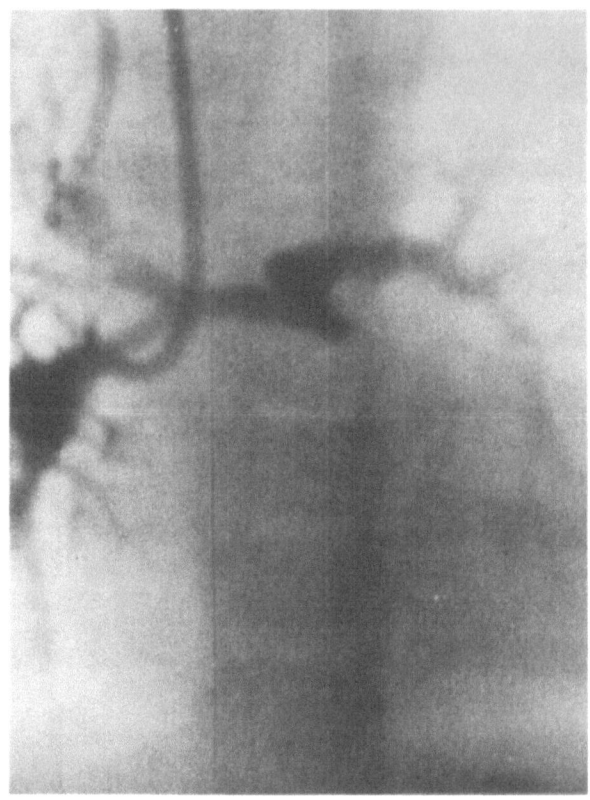

Figure 3

Fallot's tetralogy with multifocal pulmonary blood
supply. Frontal view of selective right MAPCAgram.

that unexpected post-operative pulmonary hypertension may be the
result of failure to appreciate that pulmonary supply is multifocal. This argument was based upon the study of patients with
pulmonary atresia, ventricular septal defect, and MAPCAs. In the
remainder of the lecture I hope to demonstrate that the concept
has much wider applications than this.

Continuous murmurs are characteristic of the majority of
patients with pulmonary atresia with ventricular septal defect
(Campbell and Deuchar, 1961; Ongley et al., 1966; Zutter and
Somerville, 1971). It seems probable that they are related to
stenoses either in MAPCAs, at the pulmonary end of a patent ductus
arteriosus, or in surgically constructed shunts (Macartney et al.,
1973, Macartney et al., 1974).

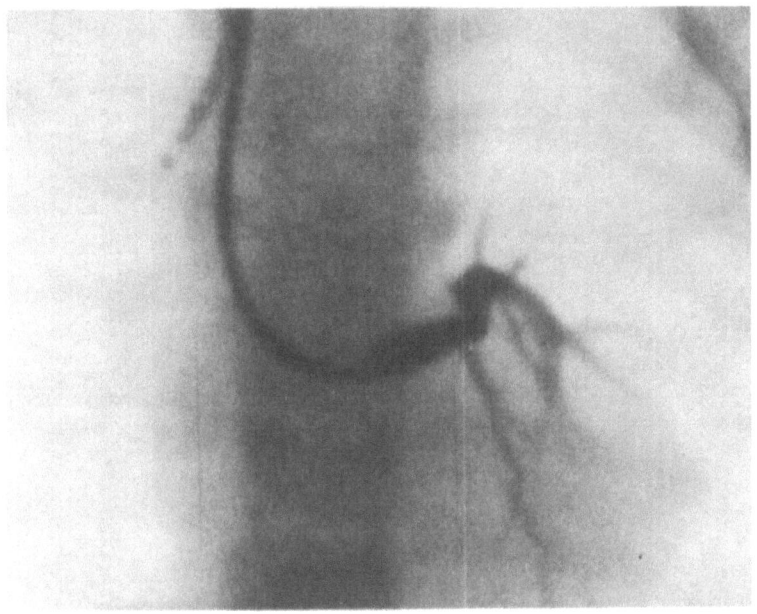

Figure 4

Fallot's tetralogy with multifocal pulmonary blood supply.
Frontal view of selective isolated left MAPCAgram.

However, continuous murmurs have also been described in
tetralogy of Fallot (Ongley et al., 1966). Apart from one patient
with a patent ductus arteriosus, these all related to other causes
of multifocal pulmonary blood supply, namely origin of one
pulmonary artery from the ascending aorta, stenosis of a central
pulmonary artery, or extensive collateral circulation secondary
to absence of one pulmonary artery or a failed surgical shunt.
We have recently investigated four patients with tetralogy of
Fallot and continuous murmurs, who do not fall into any of the
above categories. All these patients had confluent pulmonary
arteries, but exhibited MAPCAs similar in every way to those
found in pulmonary atresia with ventricular septal defect.

Three were infants, and the findings in each were surprisingly
similar. All had severe right ventricular outflow tract obstruction
and multifocal pulmonary blood supply. Figs. 2 - 4 demonstrate the
angiocardiographic findings in one such patient. In Fig. 2 a
selective outflow tract injection apparently demonstrates absence
of the right pulmonary artery. However, Fig. 3, taken from
selective injection into a MAPCA arising from the descending
aorta, shows retrograde filling of the right pulmonary artery, and

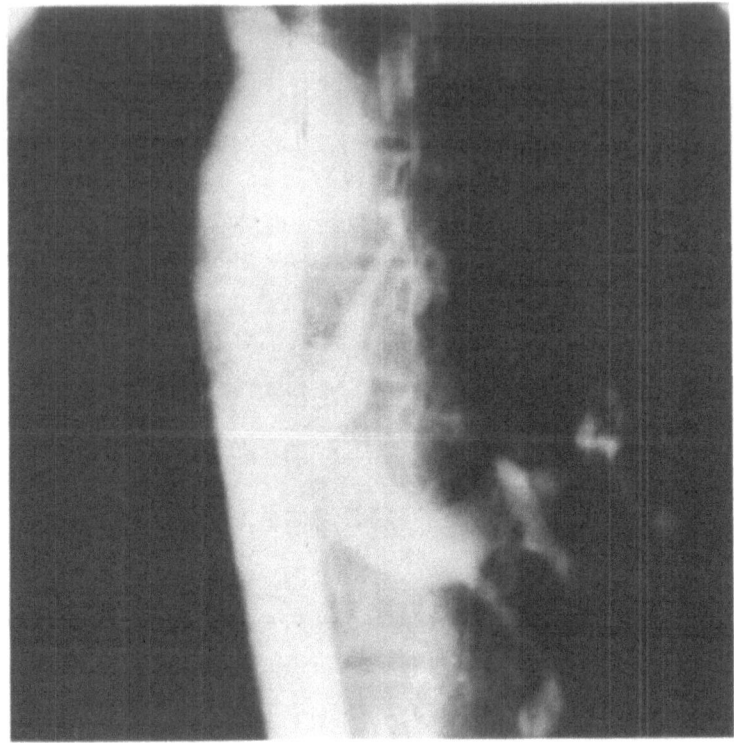

Figure 5

Fallot's tetralogy with unifocal pulmonary blood supply but
extensive collateral circulation. Frontal view of pre-operative
aortogram.

hence the main and left pulmonary arteries in a manner more
typical of pulmonary atresia. Fig. 4 shows an isolated MAPCA
filling the basal region of the left lower lobe. So this patient
has multifocal pulmonary blood supply. A similar patient died in
the immediate post-operative period from pulmonary hypertension,
having undergone radical correction of tetralogy of Fallot with
ligation of MAPCAs at the age of three-and-a-half years.

     The fourth patient is of particular interest because neither
clinical cyanosis nor cardiac failure had ever been present. A
left-sided continuous murmur was first heard at three years of
age and on investigation at the age of sixteen years, extensive
collaterals, looking in every respect like MAPCAs were demonstrated
on the left (Fig. 5). Surgery was refused on the grounds that
there was probably absence of the left pulmonary artery. However,
several years later, a left pulmonary arteriogram (Fig. 6),
demonstrated an apparently normal left pulmonary artery, except
that with the high pressure of injection, retrograde opacification

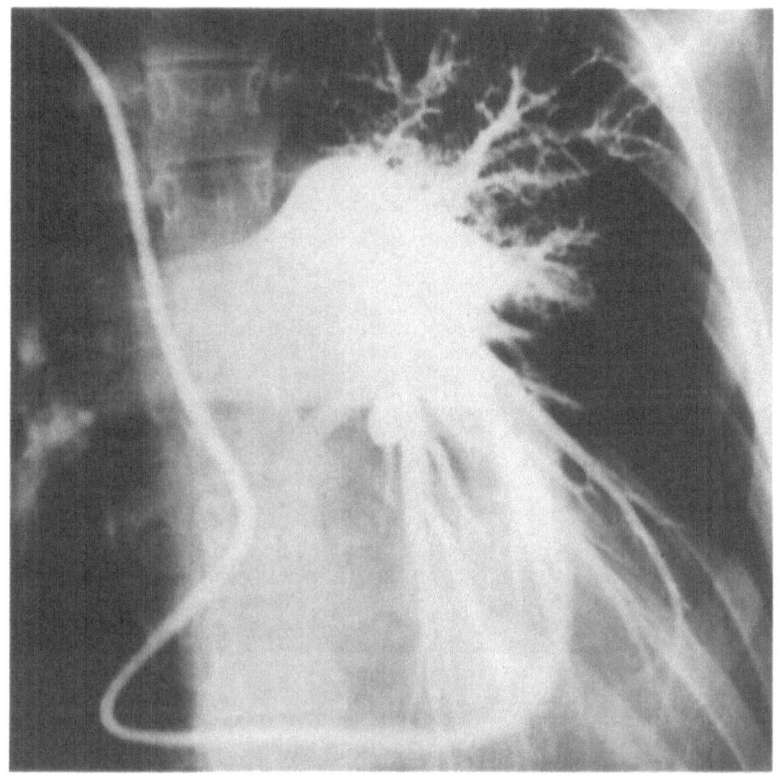

Figure 6

Fallot's tetralogy with unifocal pulmonary blood supply but
extensive collateral circulation. Frontal view of left pulmonary
arteriogram.

of the collaterals occurred in the hilar region. Through a left
thoracotomy, the MAPCA was ligated, but as there was a right aortic
arch, this was not done flush with the aorta. The patient
discharged herself before the planned radical correction could be
carried out, with the continuous murmur abolished. When she
reappeared a few months later requesting radical correction, she
was found to have developed a right-sided continuous murmur.
Aortography and selective injection into the stump of the MAPCA
demonstrated that this had sprouted an apparently completely new
branch to the right lung, anastomosing with the right pulmonary
artery immediately distal to the hilum, in the position characteristic of MAPCAs in pulmonary atresia (Fig. 7). Radical correction
was carried out without ligation of this collateral and a year
later the angiographic appearance of this vessel was essentially
unchanged.

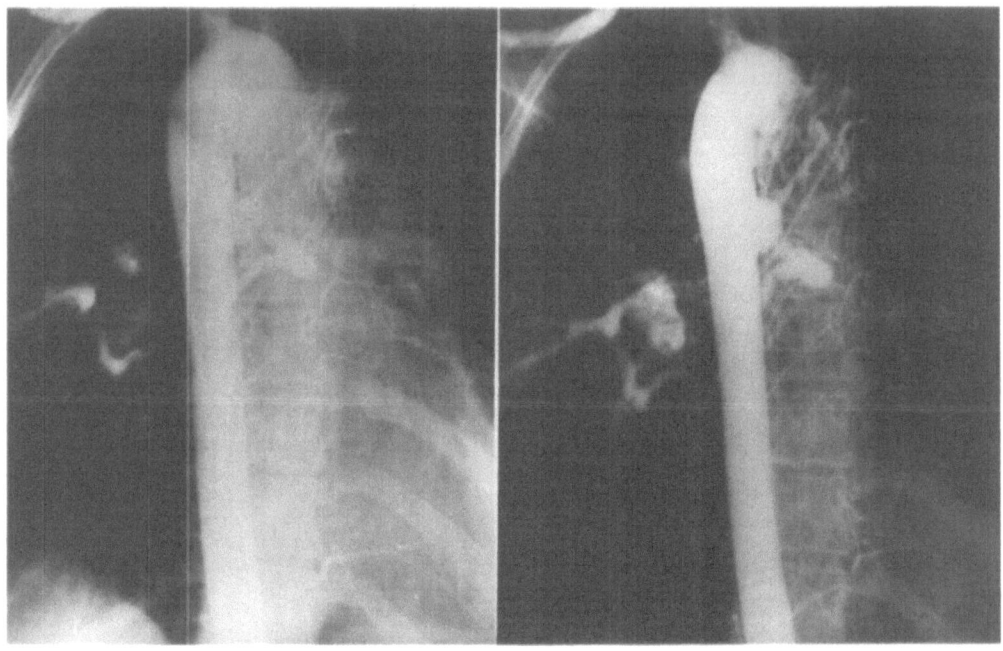

Figure 7

Fallot's tetralogy with unifocal pulmonary blood supply but
extensive collateral circulation. Frontal view of aortogram
after ligation of MAPCA (left) before radical correction and
(right) after radical correction.

Though this vessel is in a sense acquired, it bears no
resemblance to the usual acquired form of collateral blood supply,
and it seems probable that it existed as a potential channel from
early foetal life. This tentative suggestion is made in the light
of studies of acquired pulmonary blood supply in patients with
right ventricular outflow tract obstruction.

Workers at the National Heart Hospital have for some years
drawn attention to the contrast between pulmonary blood supply
in pulmonary atresia with ventricular septal defect derived from
large systemic arteries (which are MAPCAs) and small systemic
arteries, which are multiple, small, tortuous, and uncountable in

number (Jefferson et al., 1972). As we have not seen this pattern in infancy, we have concluded that it is acquired (Macartney et al., 1974). A major source of this type of collateral circulation is the intercostal arteries which almost always become enlarged in cyanotic children following a thoracotomy, on the side of the thoracotomy, no matter what type of operation has been performed. Though it is recognised that the right bronchial arteries normally originate from right intercostal arteries (Cauldwell et al., 1948; Newton and Preger, 1965) our studies of selective intercostal arteriograms in patients who have had thoracotomies indicates that the major source of collateral blood supply in these cases is from parieto-visceral anastomoses across the pleural cavity.

Fig. 8 shows an intercostal arteriogram from a patient with corrected transposition, ventricular septal defect, and pulmonary stenosis, who previously had had an end-to-side right pulmonary artery/superior vena cava anastomosis, with the proximal right pulmonary artery/superior vena cava anastomosis, with the proximal right pulmonary artery ligated. A diffuse capillary flush appeared as usual along the line of the intercostal and then opacification of pulmonary arteries and veins was faintly seen. Fig. 9 shows the same patient with one catheter introduced from the SVC into the distal right pulmonary artery, and another passed retrogradely through the aortic and left AV valves into the left atrium and right upper pulmonary vein, which has been opacified by injections of contrast medium. Because the original constriction placed at the superior vena cava/right atrial junction had slackened, distal right pulmonary artery pressure had fallen to the point at which retrograde flow from the intercostal arteries via the parieto-visceral anastomoses into the distal right pulmonary artery was occurring. The distal right pulmonary artery saturation was identical with systemic arterial saturation, whereas right pulmonary venous blood was fully saturated. This unintentional experimental model demonstrates conclusively that the systemic/pulmonary anastomoses are precapillary. Distal pulmonary arteries are only visualised in patients following injection into the intercostal arteries if there is some anatomic reason for the sixth aortic arch pressure to be extremely low. Such opacification therefore must take place in retrograde fashion and the anastomoses must be immediately precapillary. This may give rise to a haemodynamic situation which, while not strictly multifocal, may lead to the same problems of pulmonary resistance determination as multifocality.

It is well known that thrombo-embolic occlusion of small vessels in the lungs is common in cyanotic patients with polycythaemia and reduced pulmonary blood flow (Best and Heath, 1958). If such occlusions were to any extent bypassed by acquired precapillary systemic/pulmonary anastomoses, the

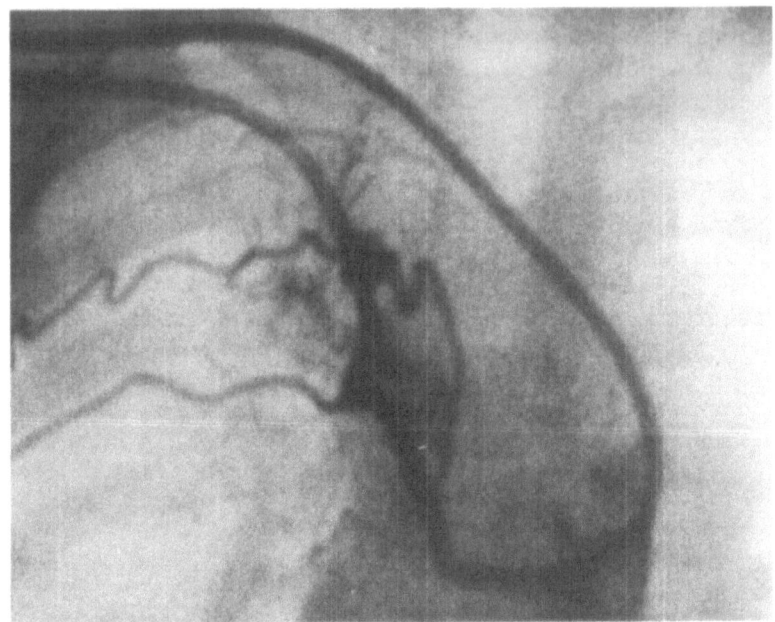

Figure 8

Corrected transposition with ventricular septal defect and
pulmonary stenosis. Previous superior vena cava/distal right
pulmonary artery anastomosis. Frontal view, selective right
intercostal arteriogram.

situation might arise in which central pulmonary artery pressure
was low pre-operatively. Total pulmonary artery flow, if based
upon central pulmonary arterial oxygen content, would be over-
estimated because of failure to allow for oxygen uptake by the
collateral circulation. After radical surgical correction the
entire systemic output would then be forced through muscular
pulmonary arteries whose resistance was in fact very high. The
haemodynamic situation is analogous to that example already given
of multifocal pulmonary blood supply with confluent pulmonary
arteries and isolated MAPCAs (Fig. 1C). We have investigated one
patient with severe tetralogy of Fallot who seems to demonstrate
this situation. Post-operatively he had severe pulmonary
hypertension completely unresponsive to pharmacological
interventions and he ultimately died of right heart failure. Both
pre-operatively and post-operatively he had evidence of extensive
acquired small collateral artery development, particularly through
intercostals. However, pre-operatively, when he had a low
pulmonary artery pressure, both pulmonary arteries and veins
opacified from injections into the aorta and intercostals. Post-

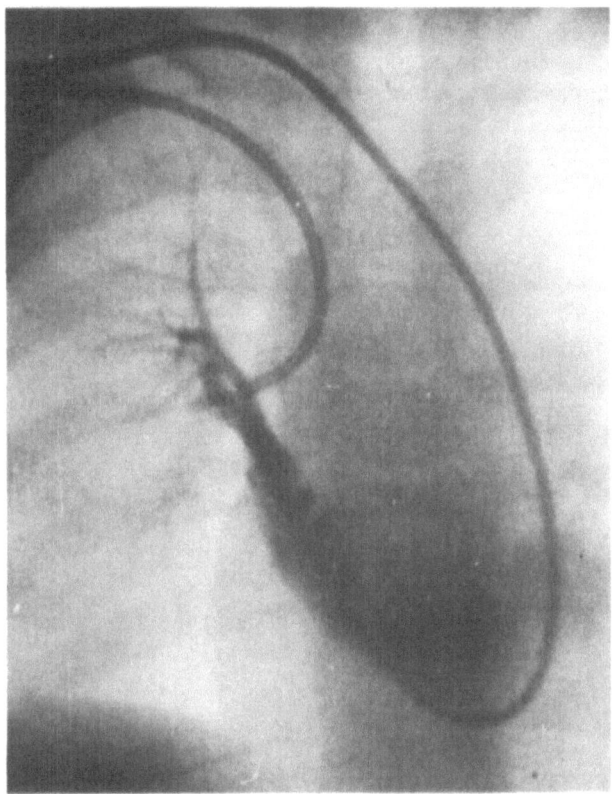

Figure 9

Same patient as Fig. 8. Frontal view, selective right pulmonary venogram. A second catheter has been passed into the distal right pulmonary artery from the superior vena cava.

operatively, the pulmonary veins alone were filled, since the pulmonary artery pressure was suprasystemic.

To sum up, the check list suggested originally for patients with pulmonary atresia with ventricular septal defect (Macartney et al., 1974) needs to be extended to any patient with pulmonary stenosis or atresia. The four basic questions are:-

1. Is either sixth aortic arch present?
2. What are the sources of pulmonary blood supply?
3. How and where do these interconnect?
4. What is the resistance to blood flow, particularly relative to the focus or foci which is to be connected to the right ventricle?

As has been indicated, the answers, particularly to the
last question, are far from completely clear as yet. I hope
that posing the questions has been worth while. It will have
been if it brings about a more critical appraisal of this
rather fundamental issue, and thereby stimulates research
directed at finding the answers.

REFERENCES

Berry, E., McGoon, D.C., Ritter, D.G., and Davis G.D., (1974);
Absence of anatomic origin from the heart of pulmonary arterial
supply: clinical application of classification. Journal of
Thoracic and Cardiovascular Surgery, 68, 119.

Best, P.V., and Heath, D., (1958); Pulmonary thrombosis in
cyanotic congenital heart disease without pulmonary hypertension.
Journal of Pathology and Bacteriology, 75, 281.

Bowman, F.O. Jr., Hancock, W.D., and Malm, J.R., (1973). A valve
containing Dacron prosthesis; its use in restoring pulmonary
artery-right ventricular continuity. Archives of Surgery, 107, 724.

Campbell, M., and Deuchar, D.C. (1961). Continuous murmurs in
cyanotic congenital heart disease. British Heart Journal, 23, 173.

Cauldwell, E.W., Siekert, R.G., Lininger, R.E., and Anson, B.J.
(1948). The bronchial arteries: an anatomic study of 150 human
cadavers. Surgery, Gynaecology and Obstetrics, 86, 395.

Chesler, E., Matisonn, R., and Beck, W. (1974). The assessment
of the arterial supply to the lungs in pseudotruncus arteriosus
and truncus arteriosus type IV in relation to surgical repair.
American Heart Journal, 88,542.

Doty, D.B., Kouchoukos, N.T., Kirklin, J.W., Barcia, A. and
Bargeron, L.M. Jr. (1972). Surgery for pseudotruncus arteriosus
with pulmonary blood flow originating from the upper descending
thoracic aorta. Circulation 45, Suppl.1. 121.

Edwards, J.E., and McGoon, D.C., (1973). Absence of anatomic
origin from heart of pulmonary arterial supply. Circulation,
47, 393.

Fabricius, J. and Rygg, I.H., (1971). Bronchospirometry in
patients with Steno-Fallot's tetralogy after palliative
operations. Danish Medical Bulletin, 18. Suppl.2. 54.

Ionescu, M.I., Macartney, F.J., and Wooler, G.H. (1972).
Reconstruction of the right ventricular outlet with fascia

lata composite graft. Journal of Thoracic and Cardiovascular
Surgery, 63, 60.

Jefferson, K., Rees, S., and Somerville, J. (1972). Systemic
arterial supply to the lungs and its relation to pulmonary
artery development. British Heart Journal, 34, 418.

Levin, D.C., Baltaxe, H.A., Goldberg, H.P., Engle, M.A.,
Ebert, P.A., Sos, T.A., and Levin, A.R., (1974). The importance
of selective angiography of systemic arterial supply to the lungs
in planning surgical correction of pseudotruncus arteriosus.
American Journal of Roentgenology, 121, 606.

Macartney, F.J., Deverall, P.B., and Scott, O. (1973).
Haemodynamic characteristics of systemic arterial blood supply
to the lungs. British Heart Journal, 35, 28.

Macartney, F.J., Scott, O., and Deverall, P.B. (1974).
Haemodynamic and anatomical characteristics of pulmonary blood
supply in pulmonary atresia with ventricular septal defect -
including a case of persistent fifth aortic arch. British Heart
Journal, 36, 1049.

McGoon, D.C., Rastelli, G.C., and Ongley, P.A. (1968). An
operation for the correction of truncus arteriosus. Journal of
the American Medical Association, 205, 69.

McGoon, D.C., Rastelli, G.C., and Wallace, R.B. (1970).
Discontinuity between right ventricle and pulmonary artery:
Surgical treatment. Annals of Surgery, 172, 680.

Newton, T.H., and Preger, L. (1965). Selective bronchial
arteriography. Radiology, 84, 1043.

Ongley, P.A., Rahimtoola, S.H., Kincaid, O.W., and Kirklin, J.W.
(1966). Continuous murmurs in tetralogy of Fallot and pulmonary
atresia with ventricular septal defect. American Journal of
Cardiology, 18, 821.

Ross, D., and Somerville, J., (1966). Correction of pulmonary
atresia with a homograft aortic valve. Lancet, 2, 1446.

Somerville, J., Barbosa, R., Ross, D.R. and Olsen, E. (1974)
(abstract). Problems of total correction after aorta to right
pulmonary artery anastomosis. British Heart Journal, 36, 399.

Zutter, W., and Somerville, J. (1971). Continuous murmur in
pulmonary atresia with reference to aortography. British Heart
Journal, 33, 905.

THE TREATMENT OF FALLOT'S TETRALOGY

DR. F. ALVAREZ-DIAZ

CARDIOVASCULAR UNIT, CHILDREN'S HOSPITAL, UNIVERSITY
HOSPITAL, LA PAZ, MADRID, SPAIN

One of the outstanding developments of cardiac surgery is the
progressive reduction in age at which total intracardiac repair of
the tetralogy of Fallot has become possible. Thus we come near to
the ideal of repairing all the symptomatic infants during the first
months of life.

Until 1970 the ideal age for total correction was over 4-5
years of age; lately this has been reduced to two years, and now
total repair is accepted after the first year of age.

The various and important factors which call for early complete
repair are:-

1.   Progressive hypertrophy of the infundibulum.
2.   Progressive fibrosis of the outflow tract and
      right ventricular myocardium.
3.   Risk of development of pulmonary hypertension
      in some cases, due to collateral bronchial
      circulation or to intrapulmonary thrombosis.
4.   Risk of neurological damage.
5.   Psychosocial trauma.
6.   Important economic and social factors.

The goal of early repair in infants will be reached by each
cardiac unit according to its capabilities. The criterion of its
methods will be its results. The results of total repair during
the first months of life should be similar to those obtained in
older children with a palliative procedure added.

MATERIAL AND METHODS

During the period from 1966 to August 1975, 416 patients with tetralogy of Fallot were operated upon at The Children's Hospital, La Paz, Madrid. Shunting procedures were carried out on 264 patients and 152 were operated on with a total correction; 87 had primary correction and 66 a two-stage procedure.

At present we perform a Waterston shunt in all patients under six months of age. Between the ages of six months and one year a Waterston shunt is used except in those cases with an anatomy favourable for total correction. Over one year of age patients with favourable anatomy undergo total correction. For those with an unfavourable anatomy (hypoplastic pulmonary arteries less than 6mm diameter, small left ventricle, and where coronary arteries cross the infundibulum) a shunt operation is done: a Waterston shunt if the patient is less than two years old, and a Blalock shunt if the patient is older.

TOTAL CORRECTION

In our series of 152 total corrections, we used conventional bypass with hypothermia to 30ºC in 100 and the Kyoto technique in two. For bypass we used 50% haemodilution and intermittent aortic cross-clamping. We use a transverse right ventriculotomy for infundibular resection and valvotomy. Closure of the VSD is done with a Dacron patch using a continuous suture with interrupted sutures in the region of the bundle of His. The atrial septum is routinely explored through the tricuspid valve and an ASD or patent foramen ovale is closed if present. With unfavourable anatomy of the outflow tract, a vertical incision is performed through the infundibulum, pulmonary ring and main pulmonary artery, extending 1cm into the left pulmonary artery. In these cases we only resect a moderate amount of infundibulum and reconstruct the outflow tract with a pericardial patch sutured with 4-0 monofilament suture. The VSD is closed as usual.

After finishing the procedure and restoring the normal circulation the caval cannulae are pulled back to the right atrium and pressures are measured in both ventricles, atria, aorta and pulmonary artery.

If the pressure index RV/LV is less than 0.75 we consider the prognosis good, agreeing with Kirklin (6). Usually in our experience, after total repair of cases with a good anatomical correction in which the outflow tract is resected without a patch, the pressure in the left atrium is 5-10mm/Hg higher than in the right atrium.

In a few cases the pressure in both ventricles is similar without a significant gradient from the left pulmonary artery to the right ventricle, and the pressure in the left atrium is high (20-25mm/Hg).

In other cases with equal pressure in both ventricles and without any gradient through the outflow tract, the pressure in the right atrium is higher than in the left atrium.

In both situations during the immediate post-operative period, the risk of development of a low cardiac output syndrome will be high. To prevent this we intensify the post-operative care, trying carefully to maintain an adequate oxygen and carbon dioxide level by mechanical ventilation, proper sedation and intra-tracheal suction for about 12 hours. Isoprenaline is given continuously to stimulate the myocardial contraction. Periodic control of the potassium level and blood volume and continuous control of arterial and left and right atrial pressures are carried out.

In 17 cases (11%) the pulmonary valve was normal without any stenosis. All of the remaining 135 cases had infundibular and valvar stenosis.

In seven cases there was an abnormal distribution of the coronary arteries which interfered with the infundibular incision. In six of these cases the total repair was possible by means of a transverse incision avoiding the coronary branch. In one case the anterior descending coronary artery was a branch of the right coronary artery crossing the infundibulum. In this case a complete correction was not possible and a Brock procedure was performed. In all cases myocardial pacemaker electrodes were implanted in order to control post-operative arrythmias.

PALLIATIVE OPERATIONS

Blalock-Taussig shunts were performed in 87 cases and no deaths occurred; all patients but one were older than six months. (Table 1).

Brock's procedure was done on 13 cases with two deaths. The first died in the operating theatre from ventricular fibrillation and the second one from severe hypoxemia during the post-operative period. (Table II).

Nine out of 164 patients operated on with the Waterston procedure died (Table III). One of them developed pulmonary oedema due to a large anastomosis; another one an acute obstruction of the fistula and the remaining cases died of hypoxemia or acute respiratory failure.

Table I
TETRALOGY OF FALLOT

Blalock-Taussig Technique   Mch.-75

ages	B-T (Soloviev)	Intrapericardial BLALOCK Mortality
0-6 Mos	1	—
6Mos-1 Yr	10	1	—
1-2 Yrs	15	7	—
> 2 Yrs	4 6	7	—
	7 2	15	—
Total	87		—

Table II
TETRALOGY OF FALLOT

Brock's Technique   Mch. 75

Ages	No.	Mortality
< 1 Yr	1	1
1-2 Yrs	6	1
2-5 "	3	—
> 5 "	3	—
	13	2 (15%)

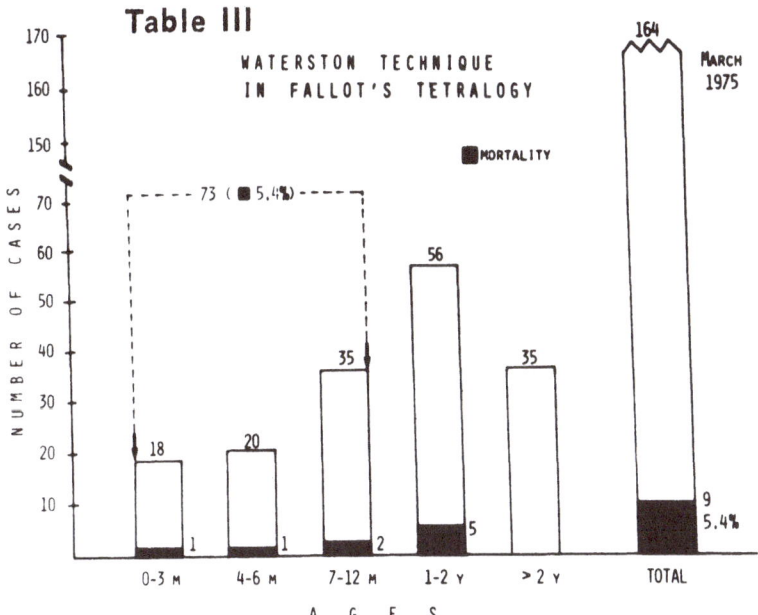

RESULTS OF TOTAL CORRECTION

There were 23 post-operative deaths in 152 patients who had total correction (Table IV). Eight were due to low cardiac output. In all of them the pressure in the right ventricle was equal or higher than in the left ventricle. In one of the post-mortem specimens a small left ventricular cavity was found. In another two complete heart block occurred. The cause of death in these cases is listed in Table V.

Atrio-ventricular dissociation presented frequently as the heart started to beat but in the majority of cases sinus rhythm was restored a few minutes later. However, six patients did not recover sinus rhythm until two to eight hours post-operatively and one did not until eight days after the operation.

A residual ventricular defect occurred in five cases. Two of them were re-operated and a small hole between two sutures was closed. The other three are well tolerated at present.

Congestive cardiac failure was present at first in almost all those cases with an outflow tract patch. All were controlled by medical treatment within 2 - 6 weeks.

DISCUSSION

Recently Barratt-Boyes (4), Subramanian (9), Starr (1),

Table IV

TETRALOGY OF FALLOT

TOTAL CORRECTION   Aug. 75

Age	No. Cases	Mortality
6 12 Mos	7	3 (42 %)
1 2 Yrs	28	7 (25 %)
> 2 "	117	13 (11 %)
TOTAL	152	23 (15 %)

Table V

TETRALOGY OF FALLOT

COMPLETE CORRECTION	August 1975

CAUSES OF DEATH

ACUTE RESPIRATORY INSUFICIENCY	2
STATUS EPILEPTICUS,CONVULSIONS	2
VENTRICULAR FIBRILLATION (Acute Coronary Insufficiency)	1
LOW CARDIAC OUTPUT	8
LOW CARDIAC OUTPUT BY LEFT HEART HYPOPLASIA .	1
LOW CARDIAC OUTPUT BY A-V DISSOCIATION . . .	2
SUDDEN DEATH	2
HEMORRHAGE	1
K$^+$ INTOXICATION	1
CARDIAC ARREST (Aspiration)	1
UNKNOWN CAUSE	1
TOTAL . . .	23

Castaneda (2) and others, have published their first cases of
tetralogy of Fallot in whom primary correction was done under one
year of age, with surface-induced deep hypothermia and circulatory
arrest according to the Kyoto University method (7). Barrett-Boyes
has reported 15 cases with a 13% mortality; Subramanian six cases
with a 33% mortality and Castaneda reports six cases without any
mortality. Total primary correction under one year of age is
preferred by these authors because of the high mortality rate
(20-30%) obtained with the shunts operations.

In our experience (3) we have four deaths (5.4% mortality)
out of 73 cases under one-year of age operated on with the
Waterston procedure (Table II). On the other hand we have three
immediately post-operative deaths from seven cases of Fallot's
tetralogy submitted to total correction below one year of age.
This represents a 42% mortality.

Accordingly our surgical preference at this time is to perform
a two-stage operation in infants under one year of age, and in our
experience the Waterston procedure affords better results than the
other palliative procedures.

The Waterston procedure is a very simple technique but is
extremely delicate. It is very easy to produce a wrong functional
shunt with an apparently good anatomical operation. Kinking of
the right pulmonary artery (8), stenosis at the anastomosis due
to excessive pulling of the right pulmonary artery (3) and
inadequate size of the stoma, are the main technical problems. The
preferential flow to the right lung in this situation is responsible
for the plethora and the interstitial pulmonary oedema that results,
leading to hypoxemia which is an important cause of post-operative
mortality. We make the incision 2-3mm long in the aorta and the
right pulmonary artery in patients under six months of age; between
six months and two years 3-4mm and over two years 4-5mm. The
resultant fistula is smaller than is usually recommended but is
still big enough to provide a good clinical result avoiding the
complications of the big fistulae, lung congestion, pulmonary
oedema and pulmonary hypertension.

Of 39 cases operated on with complete correction and previous
Waterston shunt, 20 had pre-operative catheterisation of the right
pulmonary artery, demonstrating that no pulmonary hypertension
had developed in any of them.

In our series of Waterston shunts we have a high incidence of
obstruction, which is possibly due to our tendency to produce
small fistulae. 1% developed the obstruction during the immediate
post-operative period. They were re-operated on. 6.3% were
obstructed after four to six months; they underwent a Blalock-

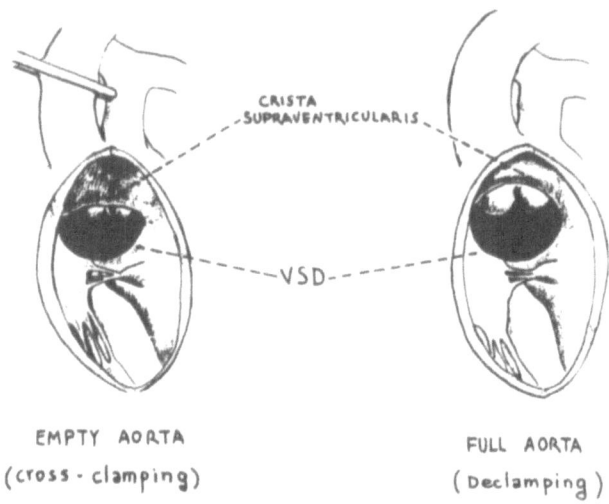

Figure 1

Good outflow tract size with empty aorta (left). Obstruction of
the infundibulum due to ballooning of the posterior wall with
full aorta (right).

Taussig shunt. 13% developed the obstruction two years after
undergoing Waterston shunt. Complete correction was performed
in these.

39 cases with a previous Waterston shunt were submitted to
complete correction. In 12 cases aortography revealed a correct
anatomy of the right pulmonary artery, and the fistula was closed
by direct aortotomy. In 13 cases the fistula was obstructed and
no repair was required. In 13 other cases the aortogram showed
some degree of kinking of the right pulmonary artery, and all of
them were repaired by taking down the anastomosis outside the aorta.

Whenever possible we try to avoid patching the outflow tract.
However, an outflow patch of pericardium was used in 53 out of
152 patients (34%). This would confirm the severity of the disease
in these patients. Using a pericardial patch we believe that the
formation of an outflow tract aneurysm is due to a significant
residual shunt or to an important residual gradient at the outflow
tract level. In our experimental unit we have implanted a 2 x 3cm
pericardial pieces in the infundibulum of eight dogs to study its
evolution. After six months in all of them the pericardium had
almost disappeared and was reduced to a fibrous scar 2-3mm wide.

The incidence of outflow tract patching according to age is as follows:- 43% below one year of age; 1-2 years 35% and over 2 years 34%.

We have observed that in some of our cases in which a good anatomical resection of the outflow tract has been performed, a significant gradient is found at the infundibular level. With the aorta cross-clamped the outflow tract had an adequate size after proper resection. With the aortic clamp off the left and right pulmonary sinuses pushed up the posterior wall of the infundibulum. The floor of the infundibulum was ballooning into the outflow tract producing a significant obstruction (Fig. 1).

Another similar situation occurred in some cases with a horizontal pulmonary artery. The excessive angulation of the pulmonary trunk at the level of the pulmonary ring in spite of its good diameter produced a significant gradient (Fig. 2).

SUMMARY

The surgical treatment on 416 patients of tetralogy of Fallot is reported. Blalock-Taussig shunts were performed in 87 patients, Brock procedures in 13, Waterston shunts in 164 and total intra-cardiac correction in 152 cases.

In view of the low mortality (5.4%) obtained with the Waterston shunt in patients under one year of age our surgical practice at this time is to perform Waterston shunts in all the symptomatic Fallots, except those cases with very favourable anatomy in which total intracardiac correction is performed. After one year of age total correction is done.

Total correction was performed in 39 cases with a previous Waterston. The way of repairing the fistula in these cases is discussed.

Two cases of functional obstruction of the outflow tract with apparently good anatomical resection are discussed.

REFERENCES

1.- Albert Starr, Lawrence I. Bonchek, and Cecile O. Sunderland; Total Correction of Tetralogy of Fallot in infancy, J. Thorac. Cardiovas. Surg. 65:45, 1973.

2.- Aldo R. Castaneda, John Lamberti, Robert M. Sade, Roberta G. Williams and Alexander S. Nadas; Open-heart surgery during the first three months of life. J. Thorac. Cardiovas. Surg. 68:719, 1974

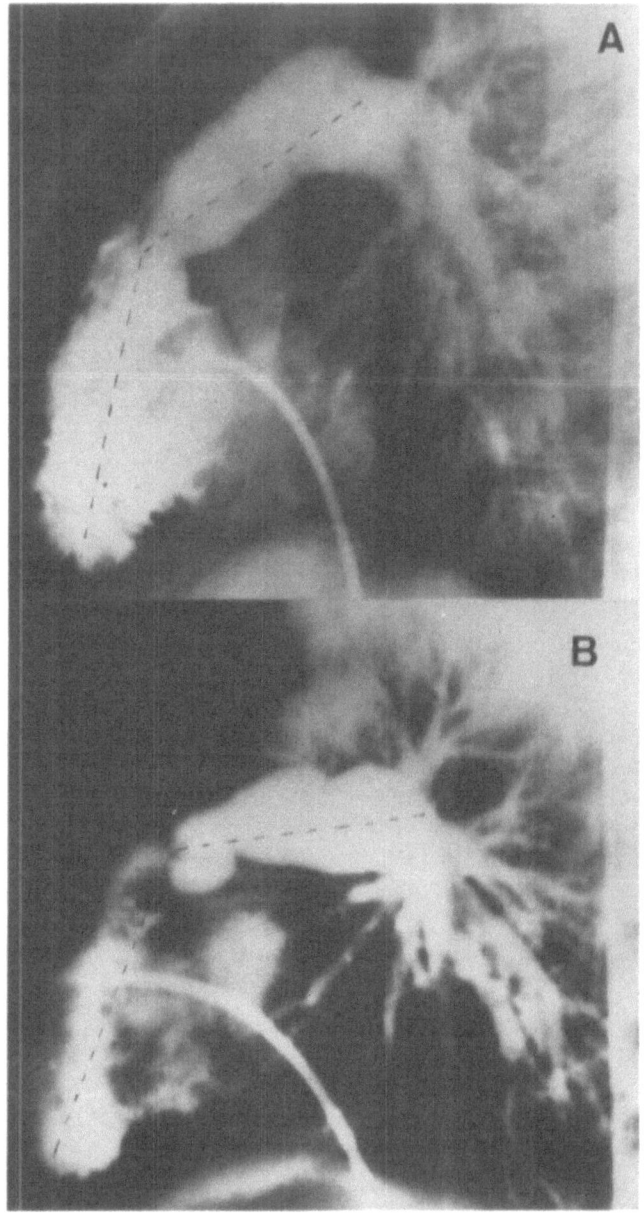

Figure 2

Compared situation of the main pulmonary artery in two cases of
Fallot's tetralogy. A. Normal. B. Horizontal position

3.- Alvarez-Diaz,F.,Brito,J.M.,Cordovilla,G.,Pérez de León,J.,
     Sánchez,P.A. and Bordiu,C.M; Ascending aorta-right pulmonary
     artery anastomosis:Waterston operation.Thorax,28:152, 1973

4.- Barratt-Boyes,B.C. and Neutze,J.M.; Primary repair of tetra-
     logy of Fallot in infancy using profound hypothermia with cir-
     culatory arrest and limited cardiopulmonary bypass:A compari-
     son with conventional two stage management.Ann.Surg. 178:406,
     1973.

5.- Francisco J.Puga,James W.Dushane,and Dwight C.McGoon; Treat-
     ment of Tetralogy of Fallot in children less than 4 years of
     age. J.Thorac.Cardiovas.Surg. 64:247, 1972.

6.- Kirklin and Karp. The Tetralogy of Fallot. From a Surgical
     viewpoint.V.B.Saunders Company, 1970.

7.- Mori,A.,Muraoka,R.,Yokota,Y.,Okamoto,Y.,Ando,F.,Fukumasu,H.,
     Oku,H.,Ikeda,M.,Shirotani,H.,and Hikasa,V. Deep hypothermia
     combined with cardiopulmonary bypass for cardiac surgery in
     neonates and infants.J.Thorac.Cardiovas.Surg.64:422, 1972.

8.- Sommerville,J.,Jacoub,M.,Ross,D.N. and Ross,K.; Aorta to
     right pulmonary artery anastomosis(Waterston's operation) for
     cyanotic heart disease.Circulation,39:593, 1969.

9.- Venugopal,P. and Subramanian,S.; Intracardiac Repair of Tetra-
     logy of Fallot in Patients under 5 years of age. The Ann. of
     Thorac.Surg. 18:228, 1974.

THE TREATMENT OF PULMONARY ATRESIA

DONALD ROSS

CONSULTANT CARDIAC SURGEON

NATIONAL HEART HOSPITAL AND GUY'S HOSPITAL, LONDON

This communication deals only with cases of pulmonary atresia with a ventricular septal defect, and here the surgical technique is not in doubt in that we aim to establish haemodynamic continuity between the right ventricle and the pulmonary arteries through a valve conduit after closure of the VSD. This manoeuvre we were first able to achieve in 1966 and the young man is alive and well approximately 10 years later.

What is in some doubt is the classification and identification of the condition, and a decision on prognosis and operability in an individual case.

A classification into four types, A B C D has been offered by Jane Somerville and although it has merit it is not particularly useful from a practical surgical point of view. What does seem to me to be important is whether a well defined pair of pulmonary arteries are present with locally derived collateral arterial blood supply or whether one or both lungs are primarily supplied by systemic vessels derived from the descending thoracic aorta. These correspond roughly to (A & B) Figure I, and (C & D) Figure 2, and offers two main sub-groups instead of four.

Confusion is added by the second group being called pseudotruncus by some clinicians and the confusion is further compounded by the synonymous use of the term truncus IV in many cases.

As pointed out by Chesler et al type IV truncus has no infundibular development detectable on angiography and no central

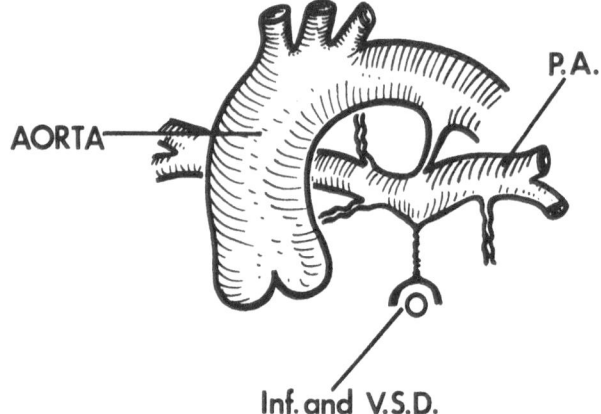

Figure 1.   Pulmonary atresia I (A + B); duct or local
            duct or local collaterals.

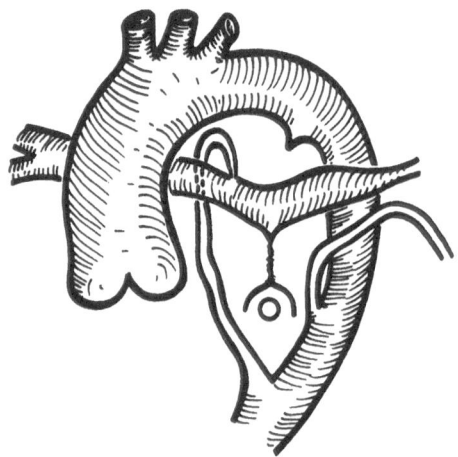

Figure 2.   Pulmonary atresia II (C + D -- pseudotruncus);
            collaterals from descending aorta.

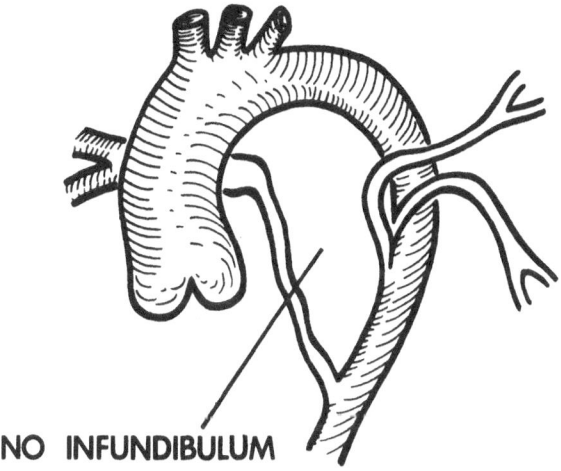

NO INFUNDIBULUM

Figure 3.   Truncus IV.

pulmonary artery remnants. All of the pulmonary blood supply is
derived from the descending aorta and the condition theoretically
inoperable by present day standards. In practical surgical terms
we could therefore regard this group of conditions as follows:

Type I
Pulmonary Atresia   -   atresia at infundibular valve, or pulmonary
                        artery level.

Type II
Pulmonary Atresia   -   with true pulmonary arteries supplied by
                        branches of descending aorta (pseudotruncus)

Type IV
Truncus   -   with no defined pulmonary arteries or
                        infundibular remnants (Fig.3)

Clinical diagnosis of the condition is dependent on an
absent outflow thrill and the presence of continuous murmurs but
an exact definition of the anatomy is dependent on angiographic
studies. In this respect late films are important since they
often bring to light unsuspected pulmonary arteries. Secondly a

descending aortogram and selective injections of the collaterals
are an essential part of the diagnosis to define the source of
the collateral blood supply (whether from local vessels, ductus
or descending aorta).

Surgical management involves either a palliative shunt
operation or the insertion of a valved conduit and this is the
one area of cardiac surgery where the biological valve has been
readily accepted, although a small minority of surgeons use a
prosthetic conduit valve.

My preference at present is for a composite conduit of
homograft and pre-clotted Dacron which offers the advantage of
sewing aorta rather than Dacron to the often extremely friable
thin distal pulmonary arteries. However the use of Prolene for
the anastomosis removes many of the earlier difficulties. The
proximal anastomosis should be countersunk as deeply as possible
into the right ventriculotomy to avoid kinking and compression
of the conduit. We have not seen the stenosis and degeneration
of the homograft conduits so dramatically described by Mavin
and McGoon except in one case previously operated upon by him.
This phenomenon must relate to their technique of graft
irradiation.

A heavy pulmonary blood flow during the insertion of the
conduit poses considerable difficulties and having used
hypothermia with circulatory arrest and its attendant neurological
and air hazards, I now find the most satisfactory technique to
be a combination of hypothermia to about 25°C plus intermittent
periods of low flow perfusion to $\frac{1}{2}$ or even $\frac{1}{4}$ the calculated flows.

Overall surgical results in 46 cases have been disappointing
and have stimulated us to try and find some explanations.
Basically the results have been moderately satisfactory in the
Type I group of patients with 24 survivors out of 36 cases but
in the pseudotruncus type of cases with one or both lungs
deriving their pulmonary blood flow from major systemic collaterals
from descending aorta the results have been bad with four survivors
out of 10 cases.

In broad terms the majority of deaths have been associated with
persistent right ventricular hypertension and pressures often
higher than those in the left ventricle. Certainly expert
anaesthetic management can pull a proportion of these children
through, and we have been impressed by the help which Rogitine
has given us latterly. Nevertheless these patients fall into
a high risk category in our hands at present.

One principle clearly enunciated by Kirklin and his colleagues

TABLE I

PULMONARY ATRESIA

46 Cases

	No.	Deaths	
Type I	36	12	33%
Type II (Pseudotruncus)	10	6	60%
	46	18	39%

TABLE   II

PULMONARY ATRESIA

46 Cases

Previous Shunts:

Waterston	23
Potts	3
Blalock	18
	44 (96%)

is to divide all the major systemic vessels arising from the
aorta at the time of surgical correction through a separate
thoracotomy. However we have not so far been rewarded by a
dramatic fall in the pulmonary vascular resistance and often
these collateral vessels are already stenosed.

Further findings at autopsy has been the presence of
thrombotic lesions in the pulmonary arterioles as described
by Rich, but these histological features are not infrequent in
many cases of severe Fallot's tetralogy dying from unrelated
causes and are not necessarily a cause of the persistent hypertension.

Certainly a majority of our cases and all the fatal cases have had previous anastomotic operations (Table II), particularly Waterston's operation and in cases of pulmonary atresia we now believe there may be special hazards in its use. We have well documented evidence that these cases usually have an increased preferential and often exclusive flow of blood to the right lung. This like the Potts' anastomosis has the effect of increasing the pulmonary vascular resistance over a period of years. Furthermore, as a result of kinking at the anastomosis no flow is likely down the left pulmonary artery since the outflow is atretic and the left pulmonary artery remains or becomes hypoplastic and contributes to the outflow resistance from the conduit.

These findings have lead us to abandon the use of the Waterston shunt in atresia cases in favour of a Blalock where a shunt is considered necessary and where a Waterston is already present we now try to operate within a year.

Finally we have recently adopted the policy of re-opening the ventriculotomy and incising the VSD patch where the right ventricular pressure ends up greater than that in the left ventricle post-operatively. This constitutes a sort of 'palliative' total correction but hopefully it will be possible to close this incision in the patch with a simple rapid suture at a later date although we have not so far reached this ideal. Also all post-operative cases studied so far show a disappointing persistence of right ventricular hypertension.

In summary correction of cases of pulmonary atresia with a valved homograft conduit is a worthwhile procedure and offers reasonable results where the pulmonary artery development is good. (Type I).

In the pseudotruncus type of case with heavy collateral from the descending aorta we try to avoid a preliminary Waterston anastomosis. Where the right ventricular pressure is persistently high post-operatively and equal to or above that in the aorta we are prepared to re-open the VSD progressively till the right ventricular pressure falls to an acceptable level.

Truncus type IV cases are avoided if possible at present by pre-operative angiographic detection of an absent infundibulum; and central pulmonary artery development.

REFERENCES

1. Somerville, J. Management of Pulmonary Atresia. 1970.
    Brit. Heart Journal. 32,641.

2. Chesler, E., Mattison R., Beck, W. Assessment of the
    arterial supply to the lung in pseudotruncus arteriosus
    and truncus arteriosus type IV in relation to surgical
    repair. 1974. American Heart Journal. 88,542.

3. Mavin G and McGoon, D.D. Re-operation after insertion
    of aortic homograft of a right ventricular outflow tract.
    1973. Annals of Thoracic Surgery, 16,122. Aug, 1973.

4. Kouchoukos, N.T., Darcia, A., Bargdron, L.M., Kirklin, J.W.
    1971. Surgical treatment of Congenital Pulmonary Atresia
    with Ventricular Septal Defect. Journal of Thoracic &
    Cardiovascular Surgery. 61,70.

5. Rich, A.R. Hitherto unrecognised tendency to the development
    of widespread pulmonary vascular obstruction in patients
    with congenital pulmonary stenosis (Tetralogy of Fallot).
    1948. Bulletin of John Hopkins Hospital, 82,389.

COMPLEX TRANSPOSITIONS AND MALPOSITIONS

P. B. DEVERALL

CONSULTANT CARDIO-THORACIC SURGEON

KILLINGBECK HOSPITAL AND THE GENERAL INFIRMARY, LEEDS

     Transposition refers to anomalies in which the great arteries
are literally transposed with respect to the morphological right
and left ventricles, i.e., the aorta rises from the right
ventricle and the pulmonary artery from the left. Throughout
this presentation the terms right and left refer to morphology
not spatial relation, except the terms "D" (dextro-) and "L"
(laevo-) which do refer to spatial position.

     Complex implies that major associated anomalies, i.e., a
ventricular septal defect or left ventricular outflow tract
obstruction, are present.

     Malposition of the great arteries implies that the spatial
interrelationships of the great arteries to each other are
abnormal, but the overall anatomy does not come within the precise
definition of transposition.

     The terms concordant and discordant refer to the inter-
relations between the atria and ventricles. The relation is
concordant when the morphological right atrium connects with
the morphological right ventricle and the left atrium with the
left ventricle. The relation is discordant when the right
atrium connects with the left ventricle and the left atrium with
the right ventricle.

     Fallot's tetralogy, pulmonary atresia and truncus arteriosus
are not considered here.

     Many complex transpositions and malposition patients have

139

been successfully treated in recent years by "corrective" surgery.
This is not to deny the importance or value of appropriately
selected palliative procedures. The optimal age for "correction"
of the complex transpositions and malpositions is undecided but
at the present time relatively few conditions can be adequately
treated in infancy.

ASSESSMENT OF COMPLEX TRANSPOSITIONS AND MALPOSITIONS

A precise haemodynamic and morphological diagnosis is necessary
when treating complex congenital heart disease. The principal
aspects of the assessment are indicated in Table 1.

A knowledge of the precise position and inter-connections of
the cardiac chambers and major venous and arterial vessels is
important. Although the details of cardiac morphology can only
be precisely defined at the time of operation, a broad plan of
action for the operative procedure should be developed beforehand.
The plan concerns the technical aspects of the perfusion and the
technique which it is hoped will be used for the corrective
procedure. This is not to deny that a flexibility of technical
approach must be maintained at the time of the operation.

Chamber and vessel localisation depends upon a combination
of invasive (e.g., angiocardiography) and non-invasive (e.g.,
bronchial tomography) techniques.

Although associated defects can be suspected on clinical
grounds, assessment requires cardiac catheterisation and
selective angiocardiography. The site and number of ventricular
septal defects must, as far as possible, be defined. Although
the morphology of a defect in a particular condition may be
predictable on a probability basis, this cannot be assumed.
Pulmonary stenosis, in complex transpositions and malpositions,
is rarely confined to the pulmonary valve alone, usually being
a more diffuse obstruction with valve, annular and subvalve
elements.

As with other congenital cardiac lesions, the level of
pulmonary vascular resistance is of major importance in
determining operability. Elevated vascular resistance is rare
with pulmonary outflow obstruction but without the latter,
pulmonary vascular disease is common with complex transpositions
and malpositions. The disease is of early onset, i.e., within
the first year of life. Transposition of the great arteries
with ventricular septal defect is the best example of a condition
in which definitive palliative or corrective surgery must be
performed before one year of age if progressive vascular disease
of the lungs is to be avoided.

TABLE I

ASSESSMENT OF COMPLEX TRANSPOSITIONS

AND MALPOSITIONS

1.   VISCERAL; ATRIAL; VENTRICULAR AND ARTERIAL POSITIONS

2.   ASSOCIATED LESIONS   V.S.D.

        PULMONARY STENOSIS

3.   PULMONARY VASCULAR RESISTANCE

4.   CORONARY ARTERIAL ANATOMY

5.   CONDUCTION SYSTEM

Coronary artery anatomy is often abnormal with complex cases.
The anatomy can often be predicted on the basis of the diagnosis,
e.g., physiologically corrected transposition, the right coronary
artery is anterior relation of the pulmonary outflow tract.
Additionally, anomalies of coronary arterial distribution, e.g.,
origin of the anterior descending coronary artery from the right
coronary artery are common. The position of the arteries can be
defined at surgery, but this is difficult, or impossible, after
previous intra-pericardial procedures. Especially in this latter
group but also in other patients, it is useful to know about the
site of major coronary arterial branches before surgery, so that
plans, e.g., the use of a valved external conduit, can be made in
advance. It is important to avoid damage to all but the very
smallest coronary arteries at surgery.

Although intracardiac delineation of the conduction system
is possible, it is a difficult technique requiring sophisticated
equipment and ideal intracardiac conditions. The site of the
conduction system in complex transpositions and malpositions is
now known with reasonable certainty on the basis of the diagnosis,
e.g., Anderson and colleagues have recently defined the position

TABLE II

COMPLEX   TRANSPOSITION

CONCORDANT ATRIO-VENTRICULAR RELATION

    i. d or l - T.G.A. + V.S.D.

    ii. d or l - T.G.A. + V.S.D. + P.S. $\begin{array}{l} \text{- VALVAR} \\ \text{- SUBVALVULAR} \end{array}$

    iii. d or l - T.G.A. + V.S.D. + P.A. BANDING

DISCORDANT ATRIO-VENTRICULAR RELATION

    i. Physiologically "corrected" transposition + V.S.D.

                                              + P.S.

                                            + V.S.D.+P.S.

                                            + A-V VALVE

of the conduction system in relation to the pulmonary outflow
tract and ventricular septal defect in physiologically corrected
transposition of the great arteries.

CLASSIFICATION OF MALPOSITIONS AND TRANSPOSITIONS (Tables II & III)

    The classification of these conditions on the basis of
concordant or discordant atrio-ventricular relations is justified
mainly since this is immediately useful in identifying the
intracardiac course of systemic and pulmonary venous return and then
in planning the operative technique, which results in that ventricle
which receives pulmonary venous return being connected to the
aorta and the systemic venous ventricle being connected to the
pulmonary artery.

There are three broad categories of corrective surgery - Table IV

    Intra-atrial rerouting of venous return always results in
the morphological right ventricle being the systemic ventricle
with one exception, i.e., anatomically corrected malposition with
a discordant atrio-ventricular relation. Here intra-atrial
rerouting of venous return results in pulmonary venous return
entering the left ventricle, which gives rise to a malposed aorta.

    Intraventricular repair alone or combined with insertion of

TABLE III

CLASSIFICATION   OF   MALPOSITIONS

(WITH   OR   WITHOUT   PULMONARY   STENOSIS)

CONCORDANT ATRIO - VENTRICULAR RELATION

    i.   DOUBLE OUTLET RIGHT VENTRICLE

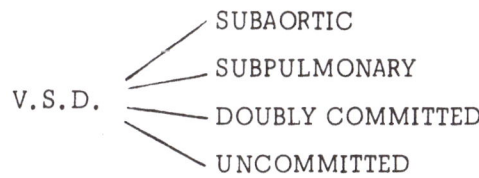

                                  SUBAORTIC

                                  SUBPULMONARY

        V.S.D.   DOUBLY COMMITTED

                                  UNCOMMITTED

    ii.   DOUBLE OUTLET LEFT VENTRICLE

    iii.   ANATOMICALLY CORRECTED MALPOSITION

    iv.   PRIMITIVE VENTRICLE

DISCORDANT ATRIO - VENTRICULAR RELATION

    i.   DOUBLE OUTLET RIGHT VENTRICLE

    ii.   DOUBLE OUTLET LEFT VENTRICLE

    iii.   ANATOMICALLY CORRECTED MALPOSITION

an external conduit usually aims to create a systemic left and
pulmonary right ventricle. The exceptions to this are
physiologically corrected transposition and double outlet right
ventricle with a discordant atrio-ventricular relation.

TECHNICAL CONSIDERATIONS OF OPERATIVE TECHNIQUES. INTRA-ATRIAL
REROUTING OF VENOUS RETURN

    Pericardium is used for the baffle and is shaped into the

TABLE IV

COMPLEX   TRANSPOSITIONS   AND   MALPOSITIONS

SURGICAL   "CORRECTION"

i.   Intra-Atrial rerouting of venous return + repair of
     associated anomalies.

ii. Intra-Ventricular repair.

iii. Intra-Ventricular repair + ventricle to pulmonary
     artery external conduit.

so-called "Trouser Patch". A 30° angle is prepared between the
limbs of the baffle and the width of the limbs is two-thirds the
circumference of the superior and inferior cavae respectively.
The waist of the baffle is measured by adding the widths of the
two limbs.

A transverse right arteriotomy is used extending the incision
posteriorly to between the upper and lower right pulmonary veins
in all but the largest right atria. The pulmonary venous atrium
is then enlarged using an oval shaped patch of woven Dacron.

The coronary sinus is not incised. The baffle suture line
is kept posterior to the sinus and does not cross the atrio-
ventricular node or bundle tissue. After baffle insertion the
coronary sinus thus drains to the pulmonary atrium.

Care is taken to avoid the sinus node tissue. It is at risk
from the superior cava cannula, superior cava tape and the upper
edge of the baffle suture line.

Every attempt is made to repair associated ventricular septal
defects via the tricuspid valve without leaflet incision. High
defects, however, require a systemic ventriculotomy, while apical
muscular defects are best exposed through a left ventriculotomy
to the left of and parallel to the anterior descending coronary
artery. Direct relief of localised left ventricular outflow
obstruction is via a pulmonary arteriotomy or through a large
ventricular septal defect.

EXTERNAL CONDUIT TECHNIQUE

After experience with irradiated and fresh antibiotic

TABLE   V

TRANSPOSITIONS AND MALPOSITIONS

INTRA - ATRIAL REROUTING OF VENOUS RETURN

SIMPLE T.G.A.

T.G.A. + V.S.D.

T.G.A. + V.S.D. + P.S.

DOUBLE OUTLET RIGHT VENTRICLE WITH SUB-PULMONARY V.S.D.

ANATOMICALLY CORRECTED MALPOSITION WITH DISCORDANT ATRIO-VENTRICULAR
RELATION

TABLE   VI

TRANSPOSITIONS AND MALPOSITIONS

INTRA - VENTRICULAR REPAIR

d - T.G.A. + V.S.D. (LARGE)

l - T.G.A. + V.S.D.

D.O.R.V. + SUBAORTIC V.S.D.

D.O.L.V.

PHYSIOLOGICALLY "CORRECTED" TRANSPOSITION

ANATOMICALLY "CORRECTED" MALPOSITION (WITH CONCORDANT ATRIA AND
                                            VENTRICLES)

PRIMITIVE VENTRICLE

TABLE VII

EXTERNAL CONDUIT PROCEDURE

(TRANSPOSITION AND MALPOSITION)

CONCORDANT ATRIO-VENTRICULAR RELATION

T.G.A. + V.S.D. + P.S.   (RASTELLI)

D.O.R.V.

D.O.L.V.

PRIMITIVE VENTRICLE

DISCORDANT ATRIO-VENTRICULAR RELATION

PHYSIOLOGICALLY CORRECTED T.G.A.

DOUBLE OUTLET RIGHT VENTRICLE

prepared aortic allografts and glutaraldehyde preserved
heterologous pericardium, the present preference is the glutaraldehyde preserved composite Dacron - Heterograft conduit prepared
by Hancock Laboratories. This is preclotted before insertion.

The conduit is inserted on the side opposite to the ascending
aorta. A vertical ventriculotomy is preferred if possible, but
ultimately this is decided by coronary arterial anatomy. Precise
tailoring of the conduit in terms of length is essential to avoid
kinking.

Application of Surgical Techniques

Tables V, VI, and VII indicate the range of conditions in
which the broad categories of surgical technique are applicable.

Transposition of the Great Arteries with Ventricular Septal Defect

This remains a difficult condition. There is great variability
in the morphology of the septal defect(s), and a marked tendency
for the establishment of pulmonary vascular disease in early life,

i.e., before one year of age. The morphology of the septal defect
is the major factor determining the choice of surgical technique.
Kinsley, Ritter and McGoon (1974) have reported successful intra-
ventricular correction when there is a very large septal defect.
A supracristal septal defect can only be adequately exposed via
a high right systemic ventriculotomy - the defect being closed so
that complete transposition is created, venous inflow then being
redirected at atrial level. As previously emphasised, multiple
or low muscular septal defects are best exposed through a left
ventriculotomy.

These considerations incline one towards a two-stage approach
to the management of infants with transposition and ventricular
septal defect, i.e., banding of the pulmonary artery in infancy,
if pulmonary hypertension is present, followed by detailed restudy
and corrective surgery between one and five years of age. This
approach, however, entails the added problems inherent in two-stage
procedures. Primary corrective surgery in infancy, though it has
its advocates (Subramanian and Wagner, 1973; Stark and colleagues,
1974) is still attended by high risks.

At this time there is, however, insufficient data to make a
clear choice between these alternative approaches and treatment
remains somewhat arbitrary and individualised. Lincoln and
Danielson and their colleagues (1972) first described the correction
of L-transposition of the great arteries with a sub-aortic
ventricular septal defect. Pulmonary stenosis was present in all
patients. An intraventricular repair creating left ventricle to
aortic continuity was achieved. Relief of pulmonary stenosis may
be complicated by the site of the right coronary artery running
anteriorly across the sub-pulmonary area. An external conduit
may be needed to bridge this area.

Transposition with ventricular septal defect and established
high resistance pulmonary vascular disease can be effectively
palliated by redirecting venous inflow but leaving the ventricular
septal defect open. Lindesmith and colleagues (1972) first applied
this approach and their conclusions have been amply supported by
subsequent experience. Four out of six such patients were dramatically
improved. There was one early death in a child in whom the
ventricular septal defect was small. In one child with transposition
and an intact ventricular septum and severe pulmonary vascular
disease, a muscular septal defect was created via a left ventriculotomy, venous inflow then being redirected. The child has done well.

Transposition, Ventricular Septal Defect and Pulmonary Stenosis

Left ventricular outflow obstruction may be due to an isolated
pulmonary valve stenosis, in which case valvotomy suffices to
relieve the obstruction. More diffuse fibro-muscular obstructions

are not amenable to local resection because of the interrelations
between the anterior mitral valve leaflet, circumflex coronary
artery, ventricular septum and conduction tissue (Shaher and
colleagues, 1967). Rastelli developed and McGoon and Wallace
(1969) applied the technique of "anatomic" correction in this
situation, in which left ventricular-aortic continuity is created
by an intraventricular patch followed by the insertion of an
external conduit to create right ventricle to pulmonary artery
continuity.

There is data to suggest that the optimal age is between
five and ten years (McGoon, Wallace and Danielson, 1973).
Treatment prior to this age is palliative. The Blalock shunt
is preferred as a technique for creating an aorto-pulmonary shunt.

Physiologically Corrected Transposition

Although the combination of a discordant atrio-ventricular
relation and transposed great arteries results in physiological
correction, most patients with this anomaly will require surgical
treatment because of associated anomalies, the main lesions being
defects of the ventricular septum, left (pulmonary) ventricular
outflow tract obstruction, "left" (systemic) atrio-ventricular
valve insufficiency and heart block.

The major recent advances in this condition have resulted
from the studies of Anderson and colleagues (1975), who have
analysed the morphology of the conduction tissue and the pulmonary
outflow tract. These workers have pointed out that, as a
consequence of malalignment of the atrial, ventricular, and conal
septa, the pulmonary outflow tract is an obliquely orientated
channel - very prone to fibro-muscular obstruction. Furthermore
the conduction tissue is an anterior relation of this outflow
tract and is related to the antero-superior margins of the left
(pulmonary) ventricular aspect of a ventricular septal defect.
The atrio-ventricular node is on the anterior aspect of the right-
sided atrio-ventricular ring (opposite to normal) and the bundle
runs from this site at the junction of the anterior atrial septum
and the base of the right atrial appendage through to reach the
anterior aspect of the pulmonary outflow tract.

In this site the conduction tissue is at risk in attempts
to relieve sub-pulmonary obstruction, while the tissue is
similarly at risk on the pulmonary ventricular side of a ventricular
septal defect.

The use of an external conduit to bypass diffuse pulmonary
outflow obstruction and closure of a septal defect via a systemic
ventriculotomy have lessened the incidence of surgically induced

complete heart block. Heart block, occurring spontaneously, remains part of the natural history of this condition.

Repair of an insufficient systemic atrio-ventricular valve is not usually successful and replacement is usually necessary. (Hallman and colleagues, 1961; Bjork and Book, 1973; and Bonfils-Roberts and colleagues, 1974). In young patients the glutaraldehyde preserved heterograft (Hancoek Laboratories) is the replacement of choice.

Primitive Ventricle

Few patients have, as yet, undergone successful partitioning of a primitive "single" ventricle. The creation of two chambers of adequate size, the effect of a prosthetic septum on "ventricular" function and the intra-ventricular connections of the atrio-ventricular valves are great problems. The site of the conduction tissue is important. It seems that if an outflow chamber is present, then the conduction tissue is similarly positioned to that in physiologically "corrected" transposition, whereas, if there is no outflow chamber, the node is normally positioned in relation to the right atrio-ventricular ring and the intra-ventricular extension of the tissue lies posteriorly.

Double Outlet Right Ventricle

Apart from the position of the great arteries and the presence or not of pulmonary outflow obstruction, the morphology of the ventricular septal defect is of major significance in determining the potential for surgical correction.

The concept of considering the defect to be committed to the aortic or pulmonary valve, or to both valves or neither, is fundamental. Thus, when there is a sub-aortic defect, left ventricle to aortic continuity can be established, (Gomes and colleagues, 1971) whereas when the defect is sub-pulmonary (Taussig-Bing Anomaly), left ventricle to pulmonary continuity is created followed by insertion of an intra-atrial baffle (Hightower and colleagues, 1969). Thomson (1967) and Kawashima and colleagues (1971) have, however, reported successful intra-ventricular rerouting of blood in the Taussig-Bing anomaly).

A non-committed septal defect is usually in the muscular septum, is of the atrio-ventricular type or is crossed by atrio-ventricular valve tissues. Each of these may preclude complete correction.

Kiser and colleagues (1968) described six patients with double outlet right ventricle with a discordant atrio-ventricular

relation and "pulmonary stenosis". All their patients and my own
had dextrocardia. Correction with or without ventriculo-pulmonary
arterial conduit insertion leaves the morphological right ventricle
serving the systemic circulation.

Double Outlet Left Ventricle

Pulmonary stenosis was present in all the patients reported
by Pacifico and colleagues (1973), but not in the original patient
of Sakakibara (1967). Left ventricle to aortic continuity is
created by intraventricular patch while right ventricle to pulmonary
artery continuity usually requires conduit insertion.

Anatomically Corrected Malposition

Isolated examples of this condition have been described.
The aorta lies anterior to the pulmonary artery but arises
normally from the morphological left ventricle. The flow of blood
is thus dependent on the atrio-ventricular relation. If this is
concordant, then surgical correction will be that of any associated
lesions. A discordant relation creates a functional situation
analogous to transposition of the great arteries, and correction
involves redirection of venous inflow.

REFERENCES

1.   Anderson, R.H., Becker, A., and Geflis, L.M.
      The pulmonary outflow tract in classically corrected
      transposition.
      J.Thor.Cardiov.Surg. 69.747.1975.

2.   Bjork, V.O., and Book, K.
      Surgical treatment of Systemic Atrioventricular Valve
      Insufficiency in Corrected Transposition. Scand.J.Thor.
      Cardiov.Surg. 7.21,1973.

3.   Bonfils-Roberts, E.A., Guller, B., McGoon, D.C., and
      Danielson, G.K. Corrected Transposition: Surgical
      Treatment of Associated Anomalies. Ann.Thor.Surg. 17.200.
      1974.

4.   Clarkson, P.M., Brandt, P.W.T., Barratt-Boyes, B.G., and
      Neutze, J.M. Isolated Atrial Inversion.
      Amer.J.Cardiol. Vol.29,877. 1972.

5.   Conti, V., Adams, F., and Mulder, D.G.
      Double-Outlet Left Ventricle. Ann.Thor.Surg. 18.402.1974.

6. Danielson, G.K., Ritter, D.G., Coleman, H.N., and DuShane,
    J.W. Successful repair of double-outlet right ventricle
    with transposition of the great arteries (aorta anterior
    and to the left), pulmonary stenosis, and subaortic
    ventricular septal defect. J.Thor.Cardiov.Surg. 63.741.1972.

7. Deverall, P.B., Bargeron, L.M. Jr., Barcia, A., and
    Kirklin, J.W. Transposition of the Great Arteries and
    Pulmonary Stenosis. Natural History and Progress in
    Treatment of Congenital Heart Defects: Edited by Kidd and
    Keith. P.175.1971. Published by Charles C. Thomas.

8. Gomes, M.M.R., Weidman, W.H., McGoon, D.C., Danielson, G.K.
    Double-Outlet Right Ventricle without Pulmonic Stenosis.
    Circ.43.Suppl.1. 31.1971.

9. Gomes, M.M.R., Weidman, W.H., McGoon, D.C., Danielson, G.K.
    Double-Outlet Right Ventricle with Pulmonic Stenosis.
    Circ.43.889,1971.

10. Goor, D.A., and Edwards, J.E.
    The Spectrum of Transposition of the Great Arteries - with
    specific reference to development anatomy of the conus.
    Circ.48.406.1973.

11. Hallman, G.L., Gill, S.S., Bloodwell, R.D., McNamara, D.G.,
    Latson, J.R., Leachman, R.D., and Cooley, D.A.
    Surgical treatment of cardiac defects associated with
    corrected transposition of the great vessels.
    Circ. 35.Suppl.1 - 133.1961.

12. Hightower, B.M., Barcia, A., Bargeron, L.M., and Kirklin,
    J.W. Double-Outlet Right Ventricle with Transposed Great
    Arteries and Subpulmonary Ventricular Septal Defect.
    Circ.39.Suppl.1. 207.1969.

13. Idriss, F.S., Aubert, J., Milton, P., Nikaidoh, H., Lev, M.,
    and Newfeld, E.A.
    Transposition of the great vessels with ventricular septal
    defect.
    J.Thor.Cardiov.Surg. 68.732.1974.

14. Imamura, E.S., Morikawa, T., Tatsuno, K., Konno, S.,
    Arai, T., and Sakakibara, S.
    Surgical considerations of Ventricular Septal Defect
    associated with complete transposition of the Great
    Arteries and Pulmonary Stenosis - with special reference
    to the Rastelli Operation.
    Circ.44.914.1971.

15.   Kinsley, R.H., Ritter, D.G., and McGoon, D.C.
      The Surgical Repair of Positional Anomalies of the
      Conotruncus.
      J.Thor.Cardiov.Surg. 67.395.1974.

16.   Kirkin, J.W., Barcia, A., Deverall, P.B., Kouchoukos, N.T.,
      and Bargeron, L.M. Jr.
      Surgical treatment of complex forms of transposition.
      Br.Heart J. 33.Suppl. 73.1971.

17.   Kiser, J.C., Ongley, P.A., Kirklin, J.W., Clarkson, P.M.,
      and McGoon, D.C.
      Surgical treatment of dextrocardia with inversion of
      ventricles and double-outlet right ventricle.
      J.Thor.Cardiov.Surg. 55.6.1968.

18.   Kawashima, Y., Fujita, T., Miyamoto, T., and Manabe, H.
      Intraventricular rerouting of blood for the correction
      of Taussig-Bing malformation. J.Thor.Cardiov.Surg.
      62.825.1971.

19.   Lincoln, C. Total correction of d-loop double-outlet
      right ventricle with bilateral conus, I-transposition
      and pulmonic stenosis. J.Thor.Cardiov.Surg. 64.435.1972.

20.   Lindesmith, G.G., Stiles, Q.R., Tucker, B.L., Gallaher, M.E.,
      Stanton, R.E., and Meyer, B.W.
      The Mustard Operation as a palliative procedure.
      J.Thor.Cardiov.Surg. 63.75.1972.

21.   Macartney, F.J., Deverall, P.B., and Scott, O.
      Single (Primitive) Ventricle. Circ. In press.

22.   McGoon, D.C., Wallace, R.B., and Danielson, G.K.
      The Rastelli Operation.
      J.Thor.Cardiov.Surg. 65.65.1973.

23.   Merin, G., and McGoon, D.C.
      Re-operation after Insertion of Aortic Homograft as a
      Right Ventricular Outflow Tract.
      Ann.Thor.Surg. 16. 122.1973.

24.   Pacifico, A.D., Kirklin, J.W., Bargeron, L.M., and Soto, B.
      Surgical Treatment of Double-Outlet Left Ventricle.
      Circ. 47. Suppl. 3. 111. 1973.

25.   Patrick, D.L., and McGoon, D.C.,   An operation for
      Double-Outlet Right Ventricle with Transposition of
      the Great Arteries.
      J.Cardiov.Surg. 9.537.1968.

26. Rastelli, G.C., McGoon, D.C., and Wallace, R.B.
     Anatomic Correction of Transposition of the Great
     Arteries with Ventricular Septal Defect and Subpulmonary
     stenosis. J.Thor.Cardiov.Surg. 58.545.1969.

27. Sakakibara, S., Takao, A., Arai, T., Hashimota, A., and
     Nogi, M. Both great vessels arising from the left
     ventricle. Bull. Heart Institute, Japan. 66.1967.

28. Shaher, R.M., Puddu, G.C., Khoury, G., Moes, C.A.F., and
     Mustart, W.T.
     Complete transposition of the Great Vessels with Anatomic
     Obstruction of the Outflow Tract of the Left Ventricle -
     surgical implications of anatomic findings. Amer.J.
     Cardiol. 19.658.1967.

29. Stark, J., Leval de Marc, R., Waterston, D.J., Graham, G.R.,
     and Bonham-Carter, R.E.
     Corrective surgery of Transposition of the Great Arteries
     in the First Years of Life.
     J.Thor.Cardiov.Surg. 67.673.1974.

30. Subramanian, S., and Wagner, H.
     Correction of Transposition of the Great Arteries in Infants
     under Surface-Induced Deep Hypothermia.
     Ann.Thor.Surg. 16.391.1973.

31. Thomson, N.B.
     Complete Repair of Taussig-Bing Abnormality.
     Ann.Thor.Surg. 4.420.1967.

32. Van Praagh R., Durnin, R.E., Jockin, H., Wagner, H.R.,
     Korns, M., Garabedian, H., Ando, M., and Calder, L.A.
     Anatomically Corrected Malposition of the Great Arteries
     (S.D.L.) Circ. 51.20.1975.

33. Van Praagh R., Perez-Trevino, C., Reynolds, J.L., Moes,
     C.A.F., Keith, J.D., Roy, D.L., Belcourt, C., Weinberg,
     P.M., and Parisi, L.F.
     Double-Outlet Right Ventricle (S.D.L.) with Subaortic
     Ventricular Septal Defect and Pulmonary Stenosis.
     Amer.J.Cardiol. 35.42.1975.

DISCUSSION

CHAIRMAN: DR. P. G. ASHMORE

VANCOUVER GENERAL HOSPITAL, BRITISH COLUMBIA

CHAIRMAN: This has been a very sophisticated morning. I
hope that some of you understand enough of these things to ask
appropriate questions. While you are thinking about this, does
someone have an early question that they could ask?

MONRO: I would like to ask Dr. Diaz a question. I was
very impressed with your large numbers, and your series of
Fallot's. I think, however, you are making a lot of work for
yourself by palliating so many of these patients, and I would
like to suggest perhaps a more aggressive approach. This has
been suggested and done successfully by Barratt-Boyes and many
others. I think apart from those few cases in which the
anatomy is unfavourable the real problems only arise with the
patients under six months, and over six months the results, using
the right techniques, are now so good that I would suggest that
you stop palliating and do more total correction. What I would
really like to ask you is what method are you using on these
patients between six months and two years, conventional bypass
or hypothermia, or what?

DIAZ: We have little experience of total correction in
this age group. Usually we use moderate hypothermia, but lately
the Kyoto technique.

MONRO: May I suggest you extend it to this group of patients
between six months and two years, because if I quote you correctly
your operative mortality in the group of 35 patients between six
months and two years is 28.5%. I personally used to use bypass
with moderate hypothermia in this group, and in two patients in
whom I had done what I thought was the best repair I could, both
had low output, and I would like to ask whether you have had
experience with this. Since giving that up and using just the

Kyoto technique in the group of patients between six months and
two years in the last year ten patients have been successfully
treated, and I would like to recommend that form of treatment.

CHAIRMAN: I think perhaps we could share this discussion
a little bit because we are very fond of operating on this group
of patients and are encouraged by the sort of thing you are
talking about, Mr. Monro, and by Barratt-Boyes experience of
operating on tetralogy in these infants under a year. However,
we cannot get his results either, and perhaps Mr. Deverall or
Mr. Ross would like to comment on this.

DEVERALL: I completely agree. I think we were totally
swept away with the enthusiasm of Brian Barratt-Boyes and a few
others, and went wholeheartedly into this primary total correction
in infancy, for about 18 months or so; at the end of it we sat
back and looked at our mortality, and it was 40% and our incidence
of heart block there. I freely admit that this is probably
a reflection on us as a group, and me as a surgeon, and all the
rest of it, but I find the correction of a complex tetralogy in a
four-month old child, whatever technique of perfusion used, is a
difficult operation, and we have gone back to palliating the
little ones. Our present mortality is very similar to Dr. Diaz,
about 5%, even in the very sick ones in the first few weeks of
life, and our second stage corrective mortality is 5%, so the
cumulative mortality of a group treated in a two-stage fashion
is about 10% as opposed to 40%. That is the present state of our
view.

CHAIRMAN: Can you tell me about why you think these infants
died?

DEVERALL: Low cardiac output. I personally found that this
occurred with the deep hypothermic technique and not only in this
group. We got very worried about it, and at least one possible
explanation in our hands was that when we did everything we
thought was right, but actually measured the temperature of the
myocardium, we found that it quite rapidly comes up not to the
temperature of the perfusate, but to room temperature. Now we
have switched in small children to the Kirklin approach to this
problem; that is low flow perfusion at 26°C and local myocardial
cooling, and in the last three months it has seemed to me that
we are getting somewhere. I suspect that in our hands, our
facilities, our skills, that we were damaging the myocardium of
these little children.

CHAIRMAN: Mr. Ross, you seem to be burning with an answer.

ROSS: I am not burning with an answer, but would like to
ask Mr. Monro what they think they are achieving by doing Fallot's
tetralogy under one year. Having tried it I think it is really a
practice in surgical virtuosity. I think it is difficult to do
and will not prevent the development of pulmonary hypertension in
any way. There is a very good cogent case for closing ventricular
septal defects before pulmonary hypertension arises. This is not

the case with Fallot's tetralogy at all. Over the age of two
years it is easy to correct Fallot's tetralogy with a simple
technique. Under the one year age group it is difficult to do,
and I believe it is more difficult to do, more risky, and I do
not know what we are achieving, except self-satisfaction.

BAILEY: At Westminster Hospital Mr. Drew has in fact been
very enthusiastic about deep hypothermia, as some of you know,
and before 1973 he had already operated on twelve Fallot's
below the age of one year; again mortality was high - around 50%.
Another thing comes in on this: I have now been involved in the
late results of the survivors, and not only do you have a high
mortality rate, but later on 50% of our survivors have come to
re-operation for combinations of re-opened ventricular septal
defect, outflow tract aneurysms, and re-stenosis of the outflow
tract, and I think this is a very important concept in the long-
term when you are operating on these small children for Fallot's
tetralogy.

CHAIRMAN: Any more comments on this? Mr. Monro, perhaps
you would care to answer Mr. Ross?

MONRO: In answer to Mr. Ross's question - what I am
achieving is this. Firstly, I take Mr. Bailey's point, and I
think we can look forward to Mr. Abrams' presentation this
afternoon which is about what will happen after 15, 20, or 30
years, but I feel that if you can get as good a result as
Barratt-Boyes does then why do two operations when one will do.
I think you have got the parents to consider. Mr. Deverall
mentioned that he had something like a 5% fall-out rate for the
second operation. That is not very high, but I try to adopt
this policy not only to Fallot's tetralogy, but a lot of things.
I think that if we can do an operation, if you like, a make or
break situation, in infancy, this is much easier to deal with.
We must think of the family unit rather than have a patient who
is marginally improved at five years, and then dies at the age
of five, which is a much greater tragedy than dying at six months.
I am not necessarily recommending that this is the only way, but
those are two of the points I am trying to clear up. A rider
to that, you should only be doing it if your results are good
enough.

CHAIRMAN: One more reason for trying to do this under a
year is that I really have a great deal of trouble with the
Waterston operation, that is not my favourite way of spending
the morning, knowing that later there is a possibility of having
to reconstruct the right pulmonary artery and then fixing the
tetralogy. We cannot seem to get no mortality in our cases the
way some people can.

ROSS: Are we all assuming that these patients need an
operation and that you cannot carry them through to the age of
two years?

MACARTNEY: I doubt very much if that is the case. This is

not something we have tried, but there is another way to deal
with tetralogies, not all tetralogies, but tetralogy with
spells, and that is to treat them with Propranalol in infancy,
and then do a total correction at an older age. That is just
another approach which has not really been seriously tried by
too many people.

MONRO: Sure, but there is no question that there is a
group of patients that you cannot touch with Propranalol.

MACARTNEY: I am not disagreeing with that at all - I am
sure there will be failures, but when Mr. Monro says that he
is talking about a certain group of patients, I would like to
ask him how long he has gone on treating those patients with
Propranalol because unless you have tried treatment with
Propranalol you cannot say that you have no alternative to
surgical treatment.

MONRO: Yes, I think that is very fair, and we have tried
this particularly to get them out of the six months into a
slightly older age group, but as I said earlier, the two patients
that I lost after 18 months had had Propranalol. Now we stopped
it a week ahead, and it may be that that is not long enough ahead,
but in some of these patients you cannot stop it so long ahead.
That is one point. Getting back to the other question, I take
your point that you can go on flogging them with beta blockers,
but when you do finally have to stop them you may be making the
total correction more difficult. We give a fair trial if
indicated, and basically we are operating as Mr. Ross asked, on
the patients who would otherwise have had a palliative shunt.

MACARTNEY: Yes, I am interested in this question of
Propranalol. We never use Propranalol at all, but interestingly
Dr. Neutze at Green Lane tells me that they do not just operate
on tetralogies. A lot of them have had a trial of Propranalol
treatment and they stop Propranalol six hours before operation,
and he, a cardiologist, a hostile cardiologist, and not a surgeon,
says that they come through the operation satisfactorily.

MONRO: Let me put you straight on one thing, Dr. Neutze is
by no means hostile, and I think the results from that unit are in
large part due to his efforts.

WATSON: As another surgeon who has had a great deal of
trouble with the Waterston operation, could I ask the panel
whether they think this operation should not be performed?
Whether in fact every effort should be made to put the Blalock
operation in its place.

DIAZ: It is a very difficult operation, and must be done
very exactly. If the right pulmonary artery is not kinked and
if the anastamosis is made very small, down to 2mm, in infants
it is satisfactory.

CHAIRMAN: Mr. English, could you come in on this, what do
you think about Waterston's operation?

ENGLISH: Well, I do not do many Waterston's now, as I do

not deal with this particular age group, but I think that it is
not a good procedure. I think that the figures of Dr. Diaz's
on which he obviously spends a lot of time and care, shows he
still had 27 of 39 cases of his Waterston's having complications.

REES: Many very competent surgeons have trouble with
Waterston's anastomosis, I mean we see all these beautiful
pictures, one thing we have to remind ourselves is that flow
through the anastamosis is related to the fourth power of the
radius, and it is obviously a very small difference in size
could make a considerable difference in flow. People like
Dr. Starr, who we all acknowledge is a very competent surgeon,
has found a lot of trouble with Waterston's and he has done a
lot of total corrections in Fallot's under the age of one and
two years, and one of his points, I do not know whether this is
relative to Mr. Deverall's point about totally correcting Fallot's,
he would not totally correct Fallot's with a very small pulmonary
artery. I am wondering whether some of Mr. Deverall's were in
this group. Another point he made is that although you might
say what is the point in correcting Fallot's without a very
small pulmonary artery, there is no doubt that these patients
do run hazards of dropping dead. In Starr's series, a whole
group of patients who were not treated in this way, died in the
intervening period from spells and various infections and other
causes. Another point is that why we pushed this programme in
Oregon was that beta blockers were not available at that time.
I do not know what the situation is now, but you could not get
beta blockers in the States prior to about 1970.

ABRAMS: I would like to support the use of beta blockers
which was I think described by my colleague Dr. Singh at
The Children's Hospital, Birmingham. They have certainly proved
life-saving. Of course, you do need to keep the patient under
continuous review because as has just been pointed out, even
with beta blockers the patients can become rapidly ill. I
would also like to agree with the suggestion of using topical
hypothermia during operations. It appears to me that the heart
becomes very much better if you pour saline at $4^{\circ}C$ on them
whenever you cross-clamp the aorta, whatever temperature the
patient is when you start.

CHAIRMAN: That was something in yesterday's discussion
that I thought we might comment on, that is the place in
congenital heart surgery of topical hypothermia, because we
certainly encounter older children who have had aortic cross-
clamping who have developed low cardiac output for no obvious
mechanical reason. We have not been protecting the myocardium,
not the way you were suggesting. Would anyone like to comment
on this problem in the older child, not in the infant, but in
the older child with Fallot's tetralogy. Does anyone cool the
myocardium locally?

DEVERALL: Yes, we have slowly come round to this. We

started using, I hesitate to use the word, Schumway's technique,
local myocardial cooling about 18 months or so ago, in congenital
heart disease, particularly in the conditions I was talking about
this morning, such as double outlets, complex transpositions,
truncuses, and I found it absolutely invaluable, and the one
thing that has convinced me more than anything else, is bothering
to measure the temperature of the myocardium when I have been
using so-called effective techniques. If I might just refer
back to Ralph Sapsford's paper on myocardial preservation, one
of the two techniques in Dr. Kirklins group was this business
of four minutes perfusion at 25°C. However good your Sarns
heat exchanger is I do not believe you can conceivably get the
myocardial temperature down in four minutes, and two minutes
at 16°C as far as I am concerned is just not worth bothering
about enough to open your mouth to give the instructions to the
pump. We found it had no effect whatsoever on myocardial
temperature, and I simply do not think we should quote that
data as in any way related to the technique of effective
superficial and deep myocardial cooling that Mr. English has
talked about. Although we do not have as sophisticated a system
as Mr. English, we try to follow what he has said, and all I can
say is that we recently looked through a group of different
conditions (they are not controlled, I freely admit it), but we
have noticed a very significant drop in the frequency with which
we need to use inotropic agents post-operatively in those patients
we have achieved adequate protection of the myocardium. If you
get good protection with up to $2\frac{1}{2}$ hours bypass as we did on
Wednesday of this week, with a complex truncus, that child came
off bypass needing no drugs at all and has done beautifully, and
this is something we did not see until we started doing this. I
think Mr. Abrams is absolutely right.

ROSS: I just want to ask Mr. Deverall, is he using the
technique of cooling the whole patient as well, as Kirklin has
suggested with reduced blood flow?

DEVERALL: Yes, we cool to 28°C. We reduce the flow to
whatever is necessary to control pulmonary flow basically, but
in addition to that we cool the heart when the aorta is cross-
clamped.

ROSS: I must say I found that a most useful technique
because we are able to reduce flow to the point where you do
not need to clamp the aorta very often.

DEVERALL: I think once the aorta is cross-clamped you
must cool the myocardium.

CHAIRMAN: Any other comments on that?

GUNNING: I agree that the sub-endocardial ischaemia that
occurs in a good coronary perfusion or particularly in the
fibrillating heart when you are doing aortic valve disease is
well known. What is not so well known is that exactly the same
thing occurs in a hypertrophied right ventricle if you cross-

clamp the aorta. Endocardial electrode pacing, getting the muscle
potential, shows a very marked depression very soon after clamping
the aorta, and this persists for quite a while after you have
restored the circulation, so I think sub-endocardial ischaemia
occurs just as much in the right ventricle as in the left
ventricle, and may account for the low output situation.

CHAIRMAN: Yes, I think so too. Would anyone like to
comment on some of the more interesting, less common lesions
that Mr. Deverall presented so nicely?

MEARNS: I would like Mr. Deverall and Mr. Ross to tell us
about the search for Dr. Somerville's aortic pulmonary connections
and Dr. Macartney's MAPCAs and how technically difficult this is,
or whether this is a simple thing that we can all do, once they
are identified by cardiologists. At the National Heart Hospital
they had abnormal aortic-pulmonary connections, and in Leeds
they have MAPCAs, and I would like to know how the surgeons can
find these and whether this is a simple thing that we should all
be trying once our cardiologists can demonstrate them for us, or
is it something that is proving technically difficult, and
occasionally you cannot find them at all?

CHAIRMAN: Well, Mr. Deverall, you must be good at MAPCAs.

DEVERALL: I think you should ask Mr. Ross, as he has much
more experience than I have.

ROSS: I think the answer is simply that it is difficult to
find a MAPCA. The ones coming off the anterior surface of the
aorta are well defined and easy to find, but the local collaterals,
the ones coming down the sub-clavians, unless they are obvious,
are difficult to find.

ENGLISH: I indicated in my presentation this morning that
I think that the bilateral sub-mammary thoracotomy had advantages
for the specific situation where we have abnormal aorto-pulmonary
vessels or abnormal bronchial collateral arteries, whatever we
wish to call them, coming off the upper descending thoracic aorta,
or indeed, from the major arterial branches of the aorta. The
reason for this is that you have access to both sides of the body.
Now Dr. Kirklin's technique is a median sternotomy combined with,
usually, a left lateral thoracotomy. He does it, in fact, on the
side of the aortic arch. This only gives you access to one side
and where you have more than one of these large vessels coming
off, if you have got access to both sides this is a great
advantage. What my question to Mr. Ross is - of the ten Type 2
cases that he corrected, his pulmonary atresia with large
vessels coming from the descending thoracic aorta, how were these
vessels approached, and how many of them had concommitant combined
lateral thoracotomies with median sternotomies?

ROSS: I cannot give you the figures for that. I can say
that one of them - one of the longest surviving ones - had his
collaterals attacked through the left chest twice, and finally
through the right chest once. He had three separate operations

over a period of eight years. The others have all been since
Kirklin postulated the technique. They have all been done through
a separate lateral thoracotomy - not postero-lateral, but anterolateral - avoiding bilateral suitcase incisions.

ENGLISH: At the same time?

ROSS: At the same time.

ENGLISH: May I make one comment. First of all I think that
in these cases where you are left with a high pulmonary artery
pressure at the end of correction you have been suggesting that
this might be treated by incising the VSD to decompress the right
ventricle. An alternative hypothesis would be that if you did an
aortogram and could demonstrate that you had somehow missed one
or two major aorto-pulmonary collaterals, you could re-operate
electively within a few hours and tie them off. Now this has been
done and reported by Dr. McGoon quite recently, as a life-saving
procedure.

MACARTNEY: Yes, I think it is a very interesting point and
it is obviously something of which people do not have much
experience but I can see that that could be life-saving in that it
means the total pulmonary valve flow would be reduced and this
means that the problems of the left ventricle are reduced, however,
according to my way of thinking, it would not make a tremendous
difference to your problem of pulmonary hypertension because it
depends actually on whether the major pulmonary collateral artery
which you are talking about anastamoses with the sixth aortic arch.
If it is isolated, I cannot see it is going to make any difference
at all because you have still got the problem of too much blood
flow through too little lung. Tying off one other vessel to them
is not going to make any difference. If you have a huge vessel
going in to the pulmonary artery, into the sixth aortic arch,
which you have missed, you could tie that off and possibly have
some effect upon the pulmonary hypertension.

TURINA: There is an alternative method which we use in
Zurich. If you have got big collaterals coming out of the
descending aorta, we would make a longitudinal pericardial
incision with the heart up and then approach the aorta. I do not
know if anybody has tried this way but it has shown good results
in our hands. If there are major vessels you need an angio
in the room so that you know where to look for them and then you
find what you also need is an intubation of the oesophagus to
pull it on the side, and you can then usually find the vessels
and tie them off.

DEVERALL: It is interesting that there is a very recent
paper - from the Mayo clinic - where Dr. McGoon and his colleagues
describe this technique. In fact they do three things. They do
a median sternotomy; they open the left pleura, and say that you
can get quite a lot of them that way. You can also get round it
very easily it says, by incising the pericardium between the SVC
and the lateral margin of the ascending aorta, and Dr. McGoon

says that there has been "no great difficulty."

TURINA: If I could just ask one question. There is one cardiac method in use which has not been discussed in some places. It fell into disrepute. We still do it in Zurich in about a third of our cases, and that is the old Brock procedure, which means a trans-ventricular dilatation of the valve and punch. We had a mortality of only 4% and strangely enough, none of those cases which came later on needed a patch. We feel that this procedure is a partial connection.

CHAIRMAN: Does anyone want to comment on that; who still uses the Brock procedure?

BLESOVSKY: I still use it, particularly in the children who have cyanotic attacks under the age of one. It is a very simple procedure and it seems particularly effective in that type of anatomy, which tends to be a localised fibrous obstruction with muscle around it. I think it is the easiest of palliative operations to perform in a small child.

BAILEY: Yes, I would like to support the view. At Westminster we have an antipathy to shunt procedures of any sort and, for this reason, we do see the Brock as a palliative procedure in the very small children because the past experience has shown us that total correction has later problems and we have a slightly higher mortality - something of the order of 8% for this as a primary procedure. Two things - we also have a lower than usual incidence of having to patch the outflow tract, and we do not find a particularly higher mortality in doing a second operation because there has been a pericardiotomy or interference there. It does not seem to affect that particularly.

YATES: Just a small comment in the Brock procedure in infants. At Sheffield it was attempted in the small ones. It was attempted to apply Brock's principle, and remember, Brock's principles apply not only to infants but to children under 9Kg, and the results were not good as far as mortality was concerned. I would just like to ask the last two speakers what the weights were of their patients?

BLESOVSKY: I have done two of them aged one year and they were all very small children. The majority of them were between the ages of 4-6 months. I am sorry I have forgotten the weights but 9Kg is an enormous size.

CHAIRMAN: That is a big one - what we call a "keeper."

BAILEY: We are doing these in the first few days of life on patients and, in fact, we have been doing them on some of these atresias. On occasion, in fact, when you have that diaphragmatic communication between a small proximal main pulmonary artery and the right ventricular outflow, if you use a sharp dilator first of all, and a great deal of courage, you can in fact go through the diaphragm and you can then dilate it serially and not have any bleeding outside the pulmonary artery afterwards.

CHAIRMAN: I was hoping actually that someone was going to talk about that because from the point of view of someone doing a lot of infant surgery, that is the dirtiest outflow tract problem of all, that is the baby with pulmonary atresia and very tight stenosis and intact septum. Would anyone like to say, very briefly, how they treat that lethal condition?

DEVERALL: First of all, I would like to say how we do, or do not treat it, because I must admit, (and I think several would agree with me), there are some babies we do not treat, and this is based on our dreadful long-term follow up of these. We have one or two in whom we have done this trans-ventricular business who have had little tiny right ventricles and we have got them to survive the operation and thought how clever we were and they have not really done very well and have died six or nine months later with grossly wrecked right ventricles. I must admit that now when we see a child that has got a hypoplastic right ventricle and total pulmonary atresia and is in a dreadful state, we do not do anything, which may be totally wrong, that that is the way we feel. If they have a reasonably sized right ventricular cavity we do a trans-ventricular valvotomy, and if that achieves an adequate rise in oxygen saturation we are very satisfied. If it does not, go back and do a shunt on top of it.

Part IV

LONG-TERM FOLLOW-UP
OF OPERATIONS FOR
CONGENITAL HEART DISEASE

LONG-TERM FOLLOW-UP OF OPERATIONS FOR CONGENITAL HEART DISEASE

L. D. ABRAMS

CONSULTANT CARDIO-THORACIC SURGEON

QUEEN ELIZABETH HOSPITAL, BIRMINGHAM

Thank you Ladies and Gentlemen, and particularly the organisers of this conference for giving me this opportunity to speak. You understand I am more or less a local boy, and one of us had to say something.

Now I believe that surgery for congenital heart disease is in fact different from any other form of surgery. I cannot think of any other form of surgery where the operation is performed early in life, often very early in life, with the certain knowledge that the patients, as soon as they know about the operation, will be conscious of it for the rest of their lives. I do not believe that people will ever alter their attitude to their hearts, though time may prove me wrong. As you well know, it is not entirely a physical attitude, and many people are always conscious of the fact that if there is something wrong with their heart it might be serious, and however much you reassure them they may not entirely get over that. Not only that, other people are conscious of it too, therefore, throughout our patients' lives they may be interfered with by other people who will tell them not to do things, or refuse to employ them or not allow them to get married, or tell them they can only have nine children and not ten, or all the other things that are liable to happen to people who have had something wrong with their hearts. So the first question is, what is long-term follow up of cardiac surgery? Well, I suppose the answer to that is contained in the 90th Psalm, attributed to Moses, the span of a man's life is three score years and ten, or by reason of great strength, four score years. No author has had so long and continuous a readership or so wide a one. No author could have made a medical statement so well proved by

human experience. And here am I, at an age which is fairly
obvious, trying to tell you about the long-term follow up of
congenital cardiac surgery in the certain knowledge that no
surgeon can in his own knowledge know the answers, and it
therefore behoves us, who are of the generation that started
cardiac surgery, to lay the foundations of that knowledge for
future generations. But of course it is a very uncomfortable
situation isn't it, not knowing how your work is going to turn
out. Therefore, I suggest we need to be a little devious in the
way we go about obtaining this knowledge. Of course there is
direct follow up. This has already been indicated to you. I
can only bring the experience of 17 years of open heart surgery
before you, and compared with 70 years, that is not very much.
It is interesting that it was in 1907 that Munro suggested that
the persistent ductus arteriosus could be treated by ligation.
It was not until 1938 that Gross actually did it. So that is
the length of the world's experience of cardiac surgery for
correction of congenital defects and it is so far only half a
lifetime. However, we are fortunate because many congenital
cardiac defects remain undiscovered until relatively late in
life, and therefore we can extrapolate backwards as well as
forward and come,I think,to some useful conclusions.

The diagram is an indication of the relative frequency of
different forms of congenital cardiac disease, and most of you
I am sure are very familiar with these figures. Let us take the
easiest one first, persistence of the ductus arteriosus. I
suppose we can well say that this is a lesion we can cure, and I
am sure in the vast majority of cases this is true whatever we do.
I ligate it: I passed through a short interval of dividing it.
This was a fascinating operation but I believe an aberrance in
the history of surgery. It is not necessary and it is easier
and just as effective to doubly ligate it. Most patients appear
to become normal. They all have an improvement in their exercise
tolerance, and I have gone on ligating ductus' at various ages,
the oldest being 63, and I did that operation eight years ago,
the patient is still alive, so there is some evidence that if
you tie a ductus that the patient will survive a normal span and
lead a normal life, and many other people I am sure close the
ductus in middle age with equally gratifying results. There
are a few exceptions, and I know of one case that some 15 years
after the ligation of persistent ductus in childhood was found
to have pulmonary hypertension and went on and died of it.
Whether that had anything to do with the presence of persistent
ductus, or whether in fact it was a development of pulmonary
hypertension separately, I do not think we can tell.

Ventricular septal defect is, of course, rather a different
story. The difficulty here is that so many of our patients look

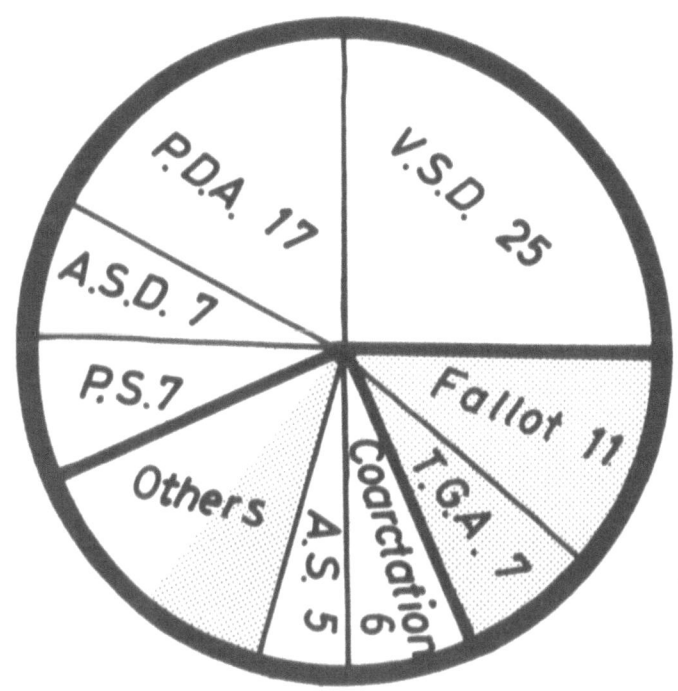

normal. The first patients I operated on with the use of cardiopulmonary bypass had ventricular septal defects operated on in
April 1958, and are alive and well today, with normal heart sounds
and normal sized hearts. We have not been able to catheterise
them, so the next question is, how do we tell that such patients
are normal? This came up yesterday in the discussion of mitral
stenosis, when somebody said they may be functioning all right,
but what is the objective evidence? Well, I would like to suggest
to you that the objective evidence we need in congenital heart
disease is the ability of the patients to live life as we understand
it. They must grow up with normal attainments, both physical and
mental, and they must do all those things other men and women do
successfully. In fact I think the most important question in
congenital heart disease the mother really asks when she brings
her daughter, and this is the usual situation we all face, is not
only what is wrong with my daughter, and what needs to be done, the
all-important question is, "Am I going to be a grandmother?"

The next question is, "Is my daughter going to be a grandmother?"
Those are the important questions, and if you remember
catheterisation studies done during delivery show that the systemic
blood pressure may approach 300 mm/Hg and it actually involves the
women concerned with quite hard physical work. I think it is
probably a better test than you can put people through on the
catheter table, even if you try very hard. I think the question
really is, will these little girls grow up, get married and have
children. All I can say about my patients with ventricular septal
defect operated on between 15 and 17 years ago, when they were
little girls, is that so many of them have grown up and had
children that I have lost count of the number of children born
to them. One interesting thing is they do not forget they have
been patients. Their obstetricians write to me and say that 15
years ago I repaired a ventricular septal defect in Miss so and so,
now Mrs so and so, and would I please come and see them to see if
they are all right. I go and see them, and I have a simple
test to see if they are all right, I say nice to see you again
Mrs. so and so, are you all right? They usually say yes. You do
the usual things of course, you listen to the chest and ignore the
systolic murmur, and you do an electrocardiogram and ignore the
R.B.B.B. The lungs look normal, and everything else looks all
right. Then she says, of course, "I do get a little tired" and
that is why you have been asked to see them. Now my personal
experience of women in pregnancy is that the ladies concerned often
do get a little tired. The trouble is that if you have had your
heart operated on that is not because you are a normal woman with
a normal pregnancy with normal symptoms, it is because you have
had your heart operated on, and that is why continuous follow-up
is so very important.

Although patients do tell surgeons that they feel well because
they do not want to disclose their horror of having an operation
in case he suggests another one, you can, I think, by judicious
questioning, find out if they are leading what you regard as a
truly normal life, and one must not stop doing this. Of course,
I am really referring to those ventricular septal defects which are
not associated with pulmonary hypertension, and if at the end of
an operation you have a pulmonary artery pressure which is below
45 or 50mm/Hg. We do not know the outlook for those patients who
have a higher pulmonary artery pressure than that at the end of
operation. Certainly quite a number of my patients are in this
situation and none of them are dead yet, but nobody seems to know
when they are going to die. What we do know is that they do not
go on dropping their pulmonary artery pressures despite having
closed the shunt. Such patients may have a degree of pulmonary
hypertension and their future is unknown.

I think the next most common lesion is atrial septal defect

and here I think perhaps I am on much firmer ground in feeling
that we know that they are going to live their proper span of
life. These of course we operate on not only when they are very
young but also much later on in life. In fact for some years I
could tell what the diagnosis was if an attractive young woman came
into my outpatient clinic wearing an engagement ring. I did not
really have to ask her the diagnosis because they were patients
with an atrial septal defect and they were going to get married
and someone had been telling them that before they got married
they should have it closed and quite right too. They were aged
between 17 and 23 then and they get married and have lots of
children and are very well, and many of them are now in their
forties and are still normal. There is one group of these that
I think is of particular interest and these are the patients with
particularly large hearts. If anybody can tell me afterwards why
some patients with an atrial septal defect have a very big heart
and some patients with atrial septal defects according to a
cardiological definition have the same size shunt and a much
smaller heart. I would be very grateful. It seems to me to be
one of the surprising phenomena of cardiology but it is true and,
not only that, some of these patients have a closed atrial septal
defect and their heart does not shrink to normal size, and this is
the group of patients about whom I am uncertain as far as their
true long-term progress is concerned. The only indication I have
of that is the follow up of these patients we operate on relatively
late in life, and typical of these is a lady I saw in follow up
last week.

   She is now 69 and says she is very well, but she has a stick
and hobbles about due to bilateral arthritis of the knees. X-ray
now looks awful. She has a heart which is certainly more than
50% of the diameter of the chest, and has great big pulmonary
arteries; in fact she was operated on in cardiac failure just under
15 years ago. She spent 12 weeks on a respirator after that. Two
weeks after she had come off her respirator, when her tracheostomy
incision had healed, she was in a two-bedded side ward when a junior
nurse happened to notice that her heart had stopped and promptly
jumped on her chest and started it again, and despite all that she
seems to have done very well indeed, being relieved of her cardiac
failure and managing to lead a normal life to a good age. So it
would appear that patients with atrial septal defect, even if they
are operated on late, have a very good outlook and can reach the
normal span of life, and I see no reason to suppose that all our
patients will not behave the same way. The follow up is longer
because some have been closed under hypothermia. I think closure
of atrial septal defect is an operation about which we can be
pretty certain, but of course I have been talking about the ostium
secundum variety and this can be extended to sinus venosus defect
with hemianomalous pulmonary venous drainage which also seems to

behave very well at follow-up. There must be uncertainties about
the behaviour of patients with ostium primium and a cleft mitral
valve. Now the trouble with this is the cleft mitral valve, and
this does, of course, make the outcome problematical.

I wish I could say something sensible about those patients
we have to operate on under the age of three years. In my
experience those are the patients who are in trouble, and often
I think they are in trouble because their mitral valves are
incompetent and this greatly increases the size of the shunt as
well as raising the left atrial pressure. One may not be able to
do a satisfactory repair. If you do do a satisfactory repair then
the evidence from our series is hopeful. We were fortunate between
the years of 1959 and 1963, that is up to 12 years ago, because we
had no mortality in a series of ostium primium with valve lesions
during that period. I say that only because that was not the
world-wide experience at that time, if I remember correctly the
collective mortality was about 17%, and even in the very good
centres it was between 12% and 15%. The other reason I say this
is that none of them have required any further surgery, in fact
none of them have even had physical signs or symptoms suggesting
that we should investigate them further, and many of them of
course have got married and become pregnant.

I am even further encouraged by the history of the single
patient I operated on in 1960 with a complete canal defect.
He was a man then of 21, and had been in bed for a year in cardiac
failure. This was not straightforward cardiac failure- he was
cachectic; he had ascites, and was permanently jaundiced. I was
asked to see him and thought I ought to try and repair this
lesion, which seemed the sensible thing to do. My senior colleague
saw him and said "I do not know what he is here for." The idea
was that he should not be allowed to die without a surgical laying
on of hands. Well of course three litres of blood ran out of his
liver into the Melrose oxygenator, and we repaired his heart and
his liver did not expand again. It was a true A-V communis
so his mitral incompetence could be seen in his scalp veins and
he did very well. He was the first patient to demonstrate
digoxin bradycardia which he suffered from for a day or two and
he needed pacing. He has since done very well. As I say, he
had been a year in bed and had only been married for 18 months,
so he had not had much of a married life. Since then he has had
three children. He is a very vigorous young man, but interestingly
enough five years ago - ten years after his operation - he developed
heart block. He has required pacing since then. It is not a
complete heart block; it is intermittent. He has a demand
pacemaker and with that he continues to lead a normal life. I
do not know whether that particular heart block is natural or
surgical. It is a little difficult over the ten years interval

to be certain, but presumably there must be some surgical scarring
in the region of the bundle, as well as natural malformation.
Heart block itself does, of course, occur as a congenital lesion
and I have very little experience of this. The longest term
patient had iatrogenic heart block. The last such patient in
which I caused this condition was in 1964 and she in fact was
eleven years old then, and when she was twelve I did her last
operation which was to fit her up with an endocardial catheter
connected to a small sized coil of the inductive system. She has
used that for nine-and-a-half years. She has grown up, married,
and had two children. She certainly turns her heart rate up to
exercise when she had the two babies, and I do not know when I will
have to operate on her next. Of course, one must remember that even
if you actually correct the defect, you may just occasionally
leave the patient with a surgical disability which is rather
unfortunate.

The next condition I would like to discuss is pulmonary
stenosis and this is a condition which I think is rather
surprising. Surprising because it is very common, perhaps that
is the trouble, it looks very simple and maybe that makes it
worse, because there is a surprising paucity of information and
literature about what really does happen to patients with
pulmonary stenosis, and there were only two papers before we
investigated the situation, both of which showed that more than
one third of the patients who had pulmonary valvotomy for valvar
stenosis finished up with impaired cardiac output response to
exercise. A very remarkable state of affairs which we did not
really believe. I thought I could do pulmonary valvotomy; I
do not think I am the only cardiac surgeon who thinks he can do
a pulmonary valvotomy. So we investigated 14 of our patients
with cardiac catheterisation at rest and exercise at varying
periods, actually between just over one and 14 years post-
operatively. Without exception they have a perfectly normal
cardiac output response to exercise so I do not know what had
happened to the patients previously reported. I would add a
rider about the nature of the operation I do. In this series
which is now rather over 100 patients, I never excise secondary
infundibular hypertrophy when doing an operation for pulmonary
valve stenosis. Of course, there are three conditions we are
discussing, pulmonary valve stenosis, infundibular obstruction,
which is of course a separate lesion, and a combination of both.
They are easy to diagnose on the angiocardiogram, and if the
patient only has pulmonary valve stenosis with secondary
hypertrophy which relaxes during diastole, I believe you should
never touch the infundibulum. The highest right ventricular
pressure I have recorded at the end of such an operation
was slightly in excess of 200 mm/Hg. That patient was
in fact operated on in 1959 as an emergency. He had a hypothermic
inflow occlusion pulmonary valvotomy. Within a few months his
electrocardiogram had resolved and he was catheterised at five

years post-operatively, when his right ventricular pressure was 35mm/Hg with a gradient of 3mm/Hg across the valve. A certain sign I think that this operation was satisfactory. The reason I stress this, is that I think this series has significantly low mortality. We have done rather more than 100 such operations on pulmonary valve stenosis ranging in age from three days to the middle fifties. Only four of them have been done in the first three weeks of life. One of those, done at three days, has had to have a second operation, which I did at the age of five years because he did have persistent pulmonary stenosis. One interesting thing about these cardiac catheterisations is that there is an excellent correlation between no gradient at rest and exercise, and very soft ejection murmur. I think we can take it that the physical signs are satisfactory, if they only have a very soft murmur. One of these patients died post-operatively when he was about three weeks old. I think that is an acceptable mortality.

The story of infundibular stenosis or combined infundibular stenosis with valve stenosis I am afraid is not so happy. I have lost one out of thirty patients, which makes it an operation of moderate danger. They also return functionally to normal and remain so over many years, and again that is a satisfactory operation.

I do not think any of us would say the same about aortic stenosis. I find this a very difficult subject, because like a lot of cardiac surgeons I am not exactly certain of the indications for operating on aortic stenosis in childhood, and my experience of operating on aortic stenosis in infancy can only be described as disastrous. It seems to me that aortic stenosis very seldom presents between the ages of one and four as a surgical problem. From the age of four onwards the results are rather better. That is we can do them as aortic valvotomies safely, and in the 20 or so cases I have done up to ten years ago, we have no operative mortality, and all I can say about them is that they have not needed another operation yet, and that I think is because so far they have not developed severe aortic incompetence, and aortic incompetence is of course a much more difficult condition to treat. It may well be that we have succeeded in our object of treating those particular patients with aortic stenosis, which is to bring them into the group of congenital aortic stenosis seen by those of us who do adult cardiac surgery. Of course, congenital aortic stenosis usually presents in the forties, fifties or even sixties and we do an aortic valve replacement for calcific aortic stenosis. I cannot tell you how long these patients can go on for; all I can tell you is that they certainly last 10 or 15 years. We are all familiar with the history after valve replacement in middle life. If the patient is fortunate enough to have sub-valvar diaphragmatic stenosis then I suppose it is more straightforward. There are not many in the series, the longest history I have is 12 years. She is very well and has no abnormal physical signs. Of course, doing this operation it is possible to damage the base of the aortic valve cusps and if that happens the outlook is different, but I would suggest that that is a condition for which we can hope for a good prognosis. It may be that supra-valvar stenosis is the same. It is a rare lesion and again the longest follow-up is 12 years. I operated on a young man with that condition. I opened his aorta vertically in the non-coronary sinus in order to get at it, and also one can of course run one's knife round the inside of the aorta, moving part of the supra-valvar ridge. He has a very satisfactory relief of stenosis. However, some of these cases as you are probably aware, have coronary ostia in the sclerotic ridge, and therefore they suffer from coronary ostial stenosis, and that is a problem which I am sure makes their outlook very problematical. This man remains well, he has a very soft murmur and does not have any other signs of recurrence of supra-valvar aortic stenosis. Since the operation he has had a daughter whom I had to operate on with supra-valvar aortic stenosis at the age of five, and she remains well five years later. That is really all I can say about that very uncertain subject.

We are on rather better ground when considering coarctation of the aorta. Many patients with established coarctation of the aorta do live for many years, as long as they do not die of cerebral haemorrhage or complications due to the associated bicuspid aortic valve. Occasionally there is rupture of the ascending aorta itself. Otherwise a lot of them do seem to live into their forties, and occasionally one sees them older than that. I say that because I think it gives us hope in considering the long-term follow up of patients who have coarctations resected whose history I think is well known to be good. The only useful thing I can say is that in common with other groups those babies on whom we operate early in life for coarctation of the aorta have a recurrence rate in our hands of 20%, which seems to be more or less the average experience, and we are now coming round to operate on them as ordinary coarctations. It seems to me that the bigger they are the better within reason when they have their second operation, and we leave them to the age of ten. My experience is that this is just as straight-forward an operation as if they had not had previous surgery.

This I think covers the majority of the defects, and I just want to say a word or two about others, these are the rare conditions, some of which we have spent considerable time thinking about and discussing this morning.

One of the more common ones is, I suppose, total anomalous pulmonary venous drainage, and here I can extract some information which is useful. I operated on a ten-year old with this condition in 1960. He has become an enormously fat man and since then is perfectly well. Obviously I got a perfectly adequate anastomosis between the common pulmonary venous trunk and the left atrium. I suppose the only question of operative success for this condition is whether that anastomosis will grow satisfactorily.

Another sort of rare condition which we have also discussed is mitral stenosis. Now I have very little experience of this condition. One patient in fact had mixed mitral stenosis and I put him in a No. 0 Starr valve the day before his second birthday, and that lasted him for 47 months and then he had signs of severe mitral stenosis. By this time he was almost six. He was quite reasonably well grown and I was surprised when I took his prosthesis out that I could put in a No. 2 Starr valve, which has a tolerable orifice I suppose for a small adult. The interesting thing I noticed about the No. 0 Starr is that the ingrowth of endothelium on the cloth had reduced the diameter in the orifice by 3mm., which is a very severe reduction indeed. He remains very well three years after this second valve replacement, and when I saw him earlier in the year and asked him how he was, he was rather quiet and did not say anything. His mother looked at me and said "He does not want to tell you how well he is in case you stop him playing football." It is only seven years improvement and it is a very problematical situation. The one patient on whom I did an open mitral valvotomy at the age of four, has done very well for nine years. In fact he is worth mentioning because I had to operate on him twice. I did an open mitral valvotomy and the valve remained competent. His immediate post-operative course was very satisfactory. However, it slowly became obvious that he was not so good. He developed a systolic murmur which became louder and louder, and I had to operate on him again. He had severe incompetence six weeks after his first operation. When I first explored his left atrium I could not see what was wrong until I looked underneath the valve and found the lateral papillary muscle to the anterior cusp was extended onto the valve cusp itself. It was the only one that did this, and I cut that papillary muscle leaving the chordae in the normal way, and he has been competent ever since. Nine years is not very long but I hope that he will continue to be competent.

Now among the other conditions I would just like to mention one of the more common of them, that is tricuspid atresia. A young lady presented to me very cyanotic at the age of 20, having had a right Blalock anastomosis done at the age of four.

She was very disabled and about to get married, so I thought I would try to do something about it, and elected to open her right chest. I found to my surprise that not only had the Blalock anastomosis stopped functioning, but the right sub-clavian artery had become a fibrous cord and the pulmonary arteries branching out distal to it into the lung were less than 2mm in diameter. The main pulmonary artery behind the vena cava was in fact of normal diameter, so I anastomosed that to the left side of the superior vena cava by doing a Glenn operation to the left lung from the right side, and ligating the superior vena cava below the anastomosis in the normal way. I did that at the end of 1966. Her palliation was good enough for her to get married and not only to conceive but to deliver a child normally by her own efforts. This really led me on to change the technique which I used for the Glenn operation.

It is not necessary to divide the pulmonary artery in order to do a superior vena cava to pulmonary artery shunt. Of course, there is less resistance in two lungs than one, and if you get an infection in one lung then you can of course shunt the blood out to the other lung, which you normally do when you get pneumonia. This operation seems to me to give an extremely useful palliation for periods in excess of seven years. Other Glenn operations I have done have been for two years longer than that and give good palliation so that at least it has been a useful operation in my hands, and no other operation of course has a history longer than this.

The other condition that I can refer to from this group of others is pulmonary atresia. The only real long-term follow up I have of a patient with pulmonary atresia also had tricuspid atresia. She was treated by direct dilatation of the pulmonary valve in the third week of life, sixteen years ago, and while I was doing that operation the bougie appeared through the back of the left atrium; that upset me considerably but did not upset the patient. She remained significantly improved by that procedure and I repeated her pulmonary valvotomy a few years later, and that became inadequate so I did a Glenn. She is moderately active, having had the Glenn operation for nine years and she has reached the age of 16 and is of normal height, certainly cyanotic and polycythaemic, and the question arises what are we doing to do next?

Now I had better turn to some of the more common cyanotic conditions. I said earlier that one of the ways one can assess function after operation is by the ordinary tests of life. Therefore, as well as doing cardiac catheterisation on people, one can exercise them in the ordinary way. For many years we have assessed the ability of our patients to climb 75' up a spiral

staircase. That enables us to assess the exercise tolerance of
our patients very usefully. This is just about all we have been
able to do to assess the function of patients with transposition
of the great arteries, which of course is another condition about
which we just do not know the answer at all. There are some ten
year follow ups. Ours only extend to eight. They are very good.
Patients have had dysrhythmias after the operation and we are in
great difficulty over extrapolating our results by reference to
any other condition - the only condition being comparable is
corrected transposition with intact septum, which of course is
haemodynamically the same condition. I understand according to
the combined European cardiologists, that this is a condition
with a bad outlook; not an immediate bad outlook, but if you take
the measurements over 20 years it does have a bad outlook.
Therefore, I feel that the outcome of the Mustard operation,
excellent though it is short term, is problematical.

This finally leaves me with the consideration of Fallot's
tetralogy, the first of which I operated on 17 years ago. Eight
of them have been operated on more than 15 years ago. The one I
operated on first had had a previous pulmonary valvotomy, and
although she survived the operation I did not do it very well,
and had to open her heart again to close a residual ventricular
septal defect and a small perforation of the base of the aortic
valve cusp. She recovered well after that third operation and
had a cardiac catheterisation 15 years after her operation.
She has, in common with fifteen other patients we have studied,
a normal cardiac output response to exercise. Their behaviour
on this particular exercise test is very satisfactory indeed.
If they are comparable in size to the member of the staff who
goes up and down the stairs with them they can equal their
performance. Some of the boys are better, the best of them
being the patient I operated on in 1959 at the age of two.
He is 6'2" tall and could beat anybody we could find in the mess,
and again he is normal on cardiac catheterisation at rest and
exercise, and the other thing about him is that in common with
five other patients he has had a cardiac catheterisation at
rest and exercise, four years and thirteen years after operation.
The interesting thing about these sequential catheterisations
is that they are all the same. That is the findings four years
after repair of Fallot's tetralogy appear in our series to be the
same as those between eleven and fourteen years after operation.
There are one or two peculiar features. One is the only
difference between the patients who have a patch across the
pulmonary valve ring and the others is that they increase their
right ventricular end-diastolic pressures on exercise slightly
more, 1 or 2mm/Hg more than the other half of patients who do
not have an outflow tract patch: that is the only detectable
difference. The other odd thing about the series is that some

of them have a supra-normal response to exercise. They do not have
as wide an arterio-venous oxygen difference as one would expect in
the normal way. That is they increase their cardiac output more
than we expect. Why this is we do not know. Of three other patients
who have also been operated on fifteen years or more ago, one is of
interest. She was operated on at the age of 22. She now has
children aged $12\frac{1}{2}$ and 10. She developed systemic hypertension
with her first baby. This is kept under control with Aldomet and
small quantities of diuretic and potassium, and she has to keep
her weight down by diet, but there has been no change in her ECG,
x-ray and physical signs over the last ten years. Another girl
also an outflow tract patch, who came up to have her cardiac
catheterisation at 14 years, when she was three months pregnant,
and so we thought we had better not do it, has been delivered of
a normal child. Of those patients operated on more than 15 years
ago, seven have children, all normal, which I think is of interest
in itself.

I have mostly stressed the history of women, because they are
the members of society who are most physically stressed during
the course of normal life, and it seems to me that we do have
some indication now that some of them may achieve their three
score years and ten. Of the men we know less. All I can say is
that the first patient who had a successful repair of Fallot's
tetralogy with an open operation in this country, is now a dental
student.

DISCUSSION

CHAIRMAN: MR. D. WATSON

KILLINGBECK HOSPITAL, LEEDS

CHAIRMAN: Well thank you very much Mr. Abrams, I think you have set us a wonderful example, having followed up your cases into adult life and beyond. Your results, in some cases quite outstanding, have raised some points. I was particularly impressed with your results for isolated pulmonary stenosis. Do I take it that you use inflow occlusion for these?

ABRAMS: Not always, no. The series is divided between inflow occlusion at normal temperature, inflow occlusion at hypothermia and bypass.

CHAIRMAN: How do you choose?

ABRAMS: I do not know how to answer that question. If I think the patient looks a comfortable physical shape to do inflow occlusion and they are not ill, that is if their electrocardiogram does not show any right ventricular strain, then I elect to do inflow occlusion at normothermia. If I think they have got very severe cyanosis then I prefer to do the operation on bypass.

YATES: I am interested in the problem of the young child with a primum lesion who has severe mitral valve regurgitation. I have had rather unsatisfactory results from my repairs in this group but very good results from patients presenting essentially as ASD secundum.

ABRAMS: I do not think the anatomy is necessarily the same. I think if you get a good result under the age of three it is because the valve happens to blow apart less, for reasons which escape me. In these patients you can fashion a decent mitral valve. Like you, I am disappointed with the results on very young patients because I think the mitral valve is often deficient. It is not just cleft, is it?

KEEN: I would like to mention two points, the first is an

advertisement for closed aortic valvotomy in the first few weeks
of life. Unlike you we have found this a very successful operation,
and we have treated five cases, the first ten years ago by closed
valvotomy in the first five weeks of life, they were all under
five weeks, with one death, and that patient had a cartilaginous
valve. The first one I saw the other day, after ten years with a
normal ECG and no diastolic murmur, and I think these valves are
as responsive to closed valvotomy in the first few weeks of life
as is the straightforward pulmonary valve stenosis. There is, I
am sure, no indication to put these young babies on bypass
because in the series I have read of, where this has been done,
the mortality has been extremely high. I share your uncertainty
about the future of the Mustard operation. We know that the
tricuspid valve stands up to systemic pressure poorly over the
years. Unrelieved pulmonic valve stenosis in middle life provokes
tricuspid incompetence. I have recently had to replace the
tricuspid valve of a corrected transposition in a patient of 16
with mitral incompetence.

CHAIRMAN: Are there any other surgeons who could claim to
understand the results of the closed aortic valvotomy?

ASHMORE: Mr. Chairman, we have a number of cases who have
inoperable cyanotic heart disease. They all want to get married,
and a number of them do, and our obstetric colleagues who are very
enthusiastic about doing abortions these days, seem to want to
abort these girls. We have now encouraged two or three of them
to go through with their pregnancies and they have really done
very well. I wonder if you have any other cases of that sort,
and what do you recommend? Do you suggest they have their
pregnancy terminated, or have you enough experience to be dogmatic
about it?

ABRAMS: I do not think I can be dogmatic, but I think that
by and large present day obstetricians view the risk of delivery
in the presence of heart disease much too seriously. I think the
experience in Dublin showed that you can be very ill with certain
valvular heart disease and be delivered safely. I would add a
proviso to that - I think they would be well advised to get
someone well used to cardiac intensive care to pop a central
venous catheter in and perhaps an arterial catheter, and monitor
their post-delivery progress very carefully. I say this because
I was asked once to do this for a patient who had aortic and
mitral valve disease. In fact the patient was so bad that the
cardiologist said could we support her circulation while she
delivers, and I said that I did not particularly want to heparinise
her while she separates her placenta. He said "Well that is a
point," so I said, "Well I will go and sit with her." I asked the
Professor of Obstetrics, whose patient she was, "How much will
she bleed." He said, "Not much," so I said, "Well, how much will
she bleed?" He said, "Not much," so I said, "Well how much will
she bleed?" He said, "A bit" so I said, "How much will she bleed?"

He said "The usual amount." I said "How much will she bleed."
He said, "Ah well, 600 to 800mls I suppose, or maybe a litre."
So I said, "All right, I will come in and watch her." I sat
by her. She delivered her baby; her venous pressure dropped
into her boots, so I transfused her and she blossomed, and I had
no trouble with her at all. It is obvious that she became gravely
ill, and I think if she had not had her blood volume looked after
she would have got into a very sticky situation indeed. You need
to keep a very careful eye on them for several days, because as
some of us know, they can go into cardiac failure after a week or
so. As far as the cyanotic ones are concerned, I do not think
they are in such a serious state as far as the exercise is concerned.
Obviously, if they are polycythemic you may have to look after
their haemorrhage problems a bit and I suggest that be done with
some care, but I think that our obstetrical colleagues ought to
be encouraged to allow women who want to have children to have
them.

BAILEY: Mr. Abrams, do you as a result of all these pregnancies,
have any information as to what the increase in congenital heart
disease is going to be as a result of our producing patients who
can have children?

ABRAMS: Yes it is a fascinating question, isn't it? The
patient I mentioned who had supra-valvar aortic stenosis is the
only child of a patient of mine I have yet seen with congenital
heart disease, although the statistics are certainly full of
gloomy prognostications. It does not look to me as though it is
going to be a very serious problem.

MACARTNEY: Just one comment, and one question, though the
comment at first may sound like a question. I do not think we
need to speculate too much about the Mustard operation, because
it looks bad enough if you do not speculate. I do not know if
you saw the long-term follow-up of the Mayo clinic Mustards.
Now they were all the best possible sort of patients to do a
Mustard on. They had a 20% late mortality in a Mustard operation.
A follow-up of 10 years maximum. 2o% late death. The question
is, you mentioned, I think quite rightly initially, the emotional
effect of heart disease, and I want to ask you a question that
flits through my mind every now and again when I am doing an
outpatients, thinking what a good doctor I am, looking after my
patients all these years, and I know you will not be able to
answer the question, but what do you think the effect is on the
patient being followed up for years? Do you think they would do
better if you just said, look, you are cured, bye-bye?

ABRAMS: Yes, I think that is a very important question. I
do, I think, have a very good answer. We did it for a bit, and
then we got into trouble because people will not employ them.
They have to come back to you and ask you to ask people to employ
them. I think that is terribly important. In fact the sequence
of events seems to me to be that you do an operation and you say

to the patient, that is perfect. You do an operation on a two-year old for closure of VSD, and then of course at $4\frac{1}{2}$ Mum comes along and says that the child is going to school in September, and what do we do about that. You say it is perfect. Then the child comes back six months later. You have written to the school doctor, of course, and they say she is now allowed to do PE and it does upset her. So you deal with that one, and then they come along when she is about twelve years old, and they say she is growing up now, and do I tell her about her periods, because, you know, I do not want to upset her heart. And then of course, a bit later on they want to know more - well you tell them they are going to grow up and get married and have children - and they say, well can she or can't she? You say, yes. Then they say, well can she get married? They come along later and say can they have children? No matter how often you do tell them these things they still come up and ask you. My feelings about the situation are now quite definite - that it is a mistake not to support them. I tell them quite straightforwardly, your daughter is normal. I want to see you again in five years time, please, because I want to know how tall you are.

CHAIRMAN: But they do need strong reassurance.

MONRO: Mr. Abrams, you said there is something like 20% re-stenosis of infant coarctation. Can I ask you whether you use a continuous suture all the way round, or interrupted, and do you think it matters?

ABRAMS: I am sure it does not matter, for a very simple reason. We had a controlled series at The Children's Hospital, Birmingham. My colleague, Mr. Roberts, does all interrupted Dexon anastamosis and I do an all continuous Dexon anastamosis, and the recurrence rate is precisely the same.

MONRO: You mentioned the treatment of tricuspid atresia with a Glenn operation. Do you have a lower age limit for the Glenn operation? I have recently run into trouble doing a Glenn in a $2\frac{1}{2}$Kg child with tricuspid atresia, and I rather wish I had done a Waterston.

ABRAMS: Yes, I would too, do a Waterston. My lower age limit is three months.

ASHMORE: You should do a Potts so that you can do a Glenn later on.

MONRO: Yes, but wait a minute, if we are going to think of the second stage treatment of tricuspid atresia, which I like to think is a Fontan procedure, we are going to get into terrible trouble with a Potts to deal with.

ASHMORE: We should not get into that, except that the results for the Fontan operations are a lot worse than for doing a Potts on one side and a Glenn on the other, and I think that is still to be proven.

Part V

CIRCULATORY SUPPORT
USING THE
INTRA-AORTIC BALLOON

CIRCULATORY SUPPORT USING THE INTRA AORTIC BALLOON

M. Terry McEnany, M.D.

Department of Surgery, Massachusetts General Hospital

Harvard Medical School, Boston, Mass.   02114

The organizers of this conference have done an outstanding job in bringing together many qualified panelists to speak on two of the most interesting and sometimes most vexing problems confronting cardiac surgeons today; conservation of the mitral valve and reconstruction of the right ventricular outflow tract. We have also heard of the many ways we can "preserve" the myocardium during cardiopulmonary bypass - each method has its forthright spokesmen and detractors. Detractors and advocates abound, also, when the subject of myocardial revascularization is raised, and it is this subject I should like to partially explore at this time. Since 1967, the most rapidly expanding aspect of cardiac surgery has been the aortocoronary bypass operation. It is estimated that, in the United States, in 1974, 50,000 patients had such a procedure performed. As the benefits of coronary artery surgery have become well documented, more and more cardiologists have begun considering the surgical treatment of coronary atherosclerosis a bona fide complement to their methods.

At the Massachusetts General Hospital, the growth of coronary artery surgery has coincided with an increasingly larger role for the intra aortic balloon in circulatory support, because of our groups' interest in the surgical treatment of the complications of myocardial infarction.[1,2] Our experience with over 500 patients who have been treated with this type of circulatory support forms the basis of this presentation.

The physiological concepts of counterpulsation as an aid to the ischemic myocardium have been investigated and substantiated for over 20 years. Kantrowitz and Kantrowitz[3] demonstrated in 1953 that coronary flow could be augmented by increasing arterial diastolic pressure. By using a pump to alternately withdraw and inject arterial blood, Clauss et al[4] were able to augment diastolic arterial pressure and reduce systolic pressure. In 1962, Moulopoulos and associates[5] reported on a balloon inserted into the descending thoracic aorta which, by displacing aortic blood, rather than pumping it, was able to achieve the same hemodynamic results and avoid the hematologic problems associated with passing blood through a mechanical pump.

The percept about which all intra aortic balloon counterpulsation revolves is that, by elevating aortic pressure during diastole, the coronary artery perfusion (driving) pressure will be increased, and, by reducing the immediate presystolic aortic pressure, left ventricular systolic pressure and ejection impedance will also be reduced. Arterial diastolic pressure can definitely be augmented by correct timing of balloon inflation according to the arterial pressure cycle. The balloon is inflated relative to the dicrotic notch of the arterial pressure wave and deflated prior to ventricular systole. This displaces 20, 30, or 40 cc. of blood from the descending thoracic aorta, increasing arterial diastolic flow and pressure. Several factors affect the degree of augmentation - heart rate, aortic/balloon volume-pressure relationship, and mean arterial pressure. In general, the higher the mean pressure, the fuller the end-systolic aorta, and the faster the heart rate, within physiologic limits, the more likely it is that there will be satisfactory diastolic pressure augmentation.[6]

Increasing the diastolic pressure does not ensure augmentation of coronary flow to the myocardium. Coronary autoregulation is not supervenable by increasing aortic root pressure. Powell and associates[7] have shown that coronary flow in normotensive, non-failing hearts is not increased by balloon counterpulsation. The coronary vasculature in ischemic areas, however, is maximally dilated and flow is solely pressure controlled. Coronary autoregulation is absent in these areas and augmentation of diastolic pressure leads to increased blood flow, increased myocardial oxygen delivery, and improved ventricular function. If diastolic pressure can be augmented without increasing the work of the heart (as with increased inotropy seen with pressor amine infusion), reduction in the area of ischemia and less progression of necrosis can be documented, as has been shown by Maroko et al.[8] Figure 1.

FIG. 1   DIFFERENCE BETWEEN EFFECT OF PRESSOR AMINE THERAPY AND THE
USE OF INTRA-AORTIC BALLOON PUMP (IABP) ON MYOCARDIAL ISCHEMIA

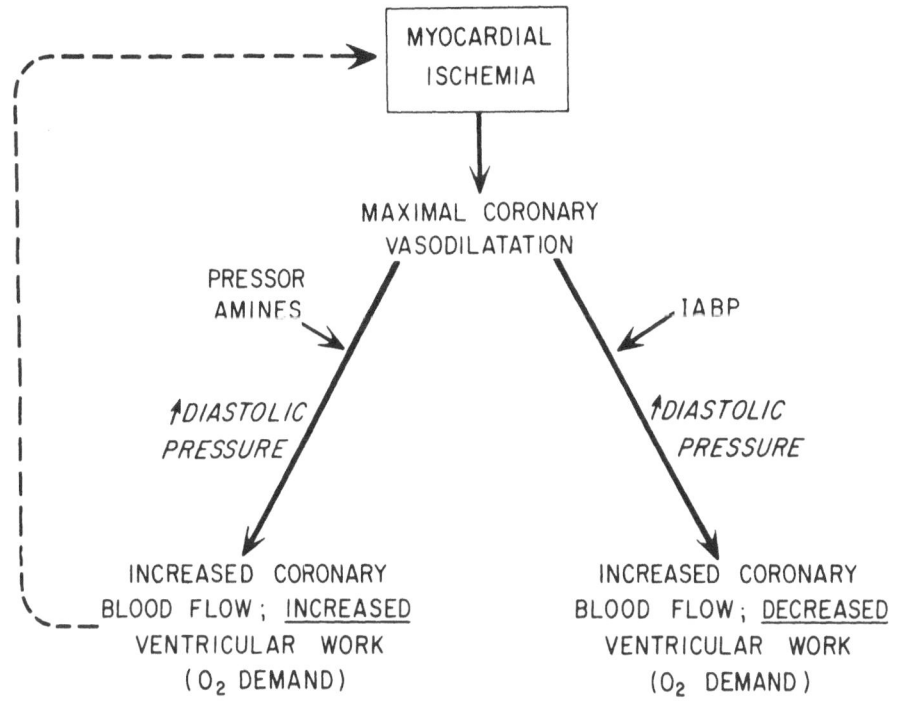

Pre-systolic deflation of the balloon aids ventricular
function by reducing left ventricular ejection impedance and
systolic pressure. Active collapse of the balloon causes the
aortic root blood to begin moving away from the heart before the
aortic valve opens, so that instantaneous systemic resistance is
greatly lowered. By this reduction in afterload, peak wall stress
is reduced along with end-diastolic volume and ventricular diameter.
This reduction in afterload leads to increased stroke volume,
reduction in end-systolic volume and an ultimate diminution in
myocardial oxygen requirements. Figure 2

The aforementioned theoretical methods of altering myocardial
metabolic supply and demand have dictated the use of the intra aortic
balloon counterpulsation device clinically for the past 8 years.

FIG. 2 EFFECTS OF PRE-SYSTOLIC BALLOON DEFLATION (SYSTOLIC UNLOADING)
ON VENTRICULAR JUNCTION AND MYOCARDIAL OXYGEN REQUIREMENTS

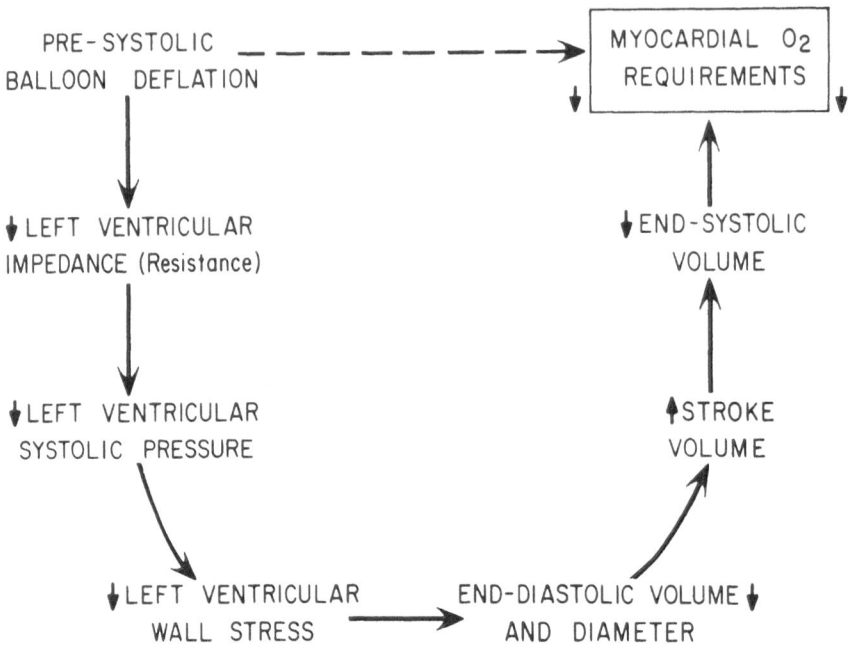

Kantrowitz et al, first used the balloon clinically in 1967,
and in 1968[9] reported treating 16 patients in cardiogenic shock
by this modality. There were 7 acute survivors. At the same time,
the AVCO-Everett Research Laboratory and surgeons at the
Massachusetts General Hospital were completing laboratory
investigation and standardization of a three-chambered intra-aortic
balloon pump which was first used clinically in November, 1968.
Buckley and associates reported the first 8 patients so treated
in 1969;[10] 4 patients survived counterpulsation, but only one
was discharged from the hospital. The low number of long term
survivors, even among those patients who responded favorably to
intra aortic balloon counterpulsation, prompted more aggressive
therapy in the hopes of increasing patient salvage.

The length of time between onset of shock and insertion of the
intra aortic balloon pump (IABP) was found to be inversely
proportional to response to the balloon, and survival. This finding
is consistent with Page and Caulfield's[11] pathological description

of necrosis of at least 40% of the left ventricular wall in all
patients dying of cardiogenic shock, and their pointing out that
the zones of necrosis were of varying age. This implied that
continued hypotension and catecholamine therapy led to expansion
of the area of ischemic necrosis over a period of days, and,
ultimately, death. Earlier balloon pumping (within 1 to 4 hours of
the onset of cardiogenic shock)[12] became the practice in the
Myocardial Infarction Research Unit of the Massachusetts General
Hospital, but the long term survivors of severe cardiogenic shock
were still few. Dunkman et al [13] reported only 4 survivors out
of the first 25 patients treated with the balloon alone at the
Massachusetts General Hospital. In 1970, Mundth [14] performed
the first successful revascularization for post-infarction
cardiogenic shock, utilizing the IABP for support during cardiac
catheterization, preoperatively, and the early postoperative
period. This success has led to a rapid growth in the use of the
intra aortic balloon as a circulatory assist device throughout the
United States.

The AVCO balloon pumping system is in use in about 300
hospitals in the United States, and about 6,000 patients have been
treated with intra aortic balloon counterpulsation. From November,
1968, through July, 1975, 506 patients have had an intra aortic
balloon inserted at the Massachusetts General Hospital. The growth
of this experience can be seen in Figure 3.

FIGURE 3

PATIENTS RECEIVING
INTRA AORTIC BALLOON PUMP COUNTERPULSATION

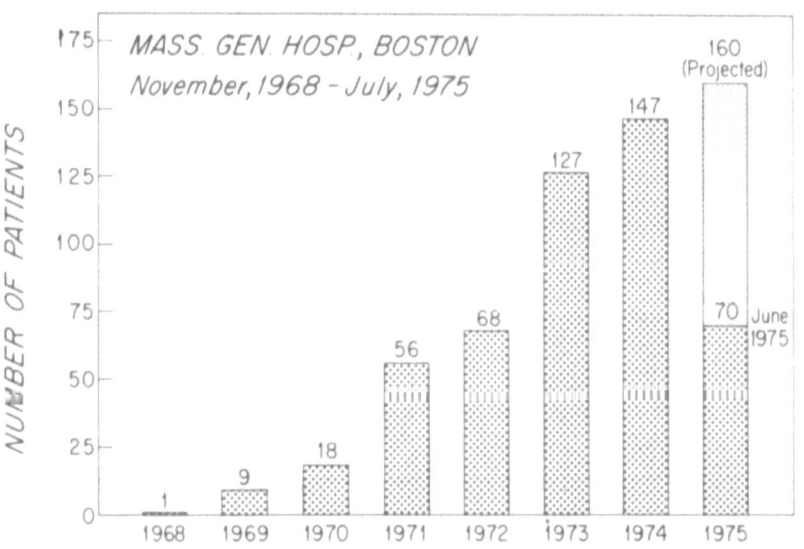

Five patients have had an IABP inserted twice; 3 of these have
survived. 399 patients have had their balloons removed. In this
group are 5 patients in whom the balloon was inserted (for
cardiogenic shock) at another hospital, the patient studied
angiographically, found to be operable, and then transferred to
the Massachusetts General Hospital for surgical treatment. Eight
patients have been so treated; 2 died in the operating room and
one expired postoperatively while still on IABP support.

The indications for intra aortic balloon counterpulsation have
expanded with time and can be seen in Table I.

TABLE I

INDICATIONS FOR IABP PLACEMENT

Post-myocardial infarction cardiogenic shock

Post-myocardial infarction pain (threatened
  extension of infarction)

Post-myocardial infarction ventricular
  irritability

Post-myocardial infarction ventricular failure
  secondary to mitral regurgitation or ruptured
  interventricular septum

Unstable angina pectoris

Crescendo angina pectoris (pre-angiography)

Post-cardiotomy cardiogenic shock

Angiographically proven main left coronary
  artery stenosis

Anteroseptal myocardial infarction in young man

Postoperative low cardiac output

Intra-operative hypotension

Post-myocardial infarction cardiogenic shock was the sole indication
for IABP support until 1971, when the balloon was inserted for post-
cardiotomy cardiogenic shock for the first time, to help wean a
patient from cardiopulmonary bypass. Buckley, Craver et al [15]
reported in 1972 on 26 patients treated by this modality, with
long term survival in 10. The use of IABP in this clinical setting
has expanded greatly and it is now standard practice for any patient
who cannot be weaned from cardiopulmonary bypass following an
operation for coronary artery disease or an aortic valve replacement.

Its effectiveness has been proven in these two instances; IABP
counterpulsation has not been successful in the rare patient with
mitral valve disease who cannot be separated from bypass, because
of severe pulmonary hypertension or diffuse ventricular dysfunction.
Our philosophy with the use of the balloon in the operating room
is that if there has been an identifiable cardiac insult, i.e.
intra-operative myocardial infarction or prolonged global anoxia
leading to subendocardial ischemia/necrosis, which is hindering
effective cardiac action and which, if the patient can be
supported for several days, is compatible with long term survival,
insertion of the IABP is indicated to improve myocardial collateral
flow and contribute to reduced oxygen demands of the remaining
viable myocardium. The recent exposition of the detrimental effects
of pressor amines on subendocardial coronary perfusion [16] has
led Phillips et al [17] to utilize the calculated reduction in
subendocardial perfusion, expressed as a reduced endocardial
viability ratio (EVR), a statement of DPTI:TTI ratio, [18] as an
indicator for the use of the intra aortic balloon in the absence
of clinical cardiogenic shock, in order to avoid pressor medications.
This may well be a justification of even increased IABP use in the
future.

As IABP experience accumulated in patients with cardiogenic
shock, the results of reduction in myocardial ischemia became more
impressive to clinicians involved with balloon counterpulsation.
Reduction of electrocardiographic evidence of ischemia, with
lowering of ST segment elevations and diminution of frequency of
ventricular extra systoles, as well as the control of unrelenting
ischemic coronary pain became commonplace. With increased surgical
experience and confidence in the technical aspects of balloon
counterpulsation, the indications for its use expanded.

In 1972, Maroko et al [8] presented two patients with marked
(up to 80%) decrease in ΣST (sum of ST elevations) and NST
(number of sites with S-T segment elevation exceeding 0.1 mm) with
balloon pumping after myocardial infarction. In the hopes of
reducing the size of acute myocardial infarctions, we have inserted
the balloon in 11 young (under 50 years old) males with acute
anteroseptal myocardial infarctions. Decrease in ΣST has been
demonstrable in all patients, all have survived, and there have
been no complications related to the intra aortic balloon in these
patients.

Reversing the acute ischemia in patients with pre-infarction
angina pectoris has been an especially useful indication for balloon
pumping. 42 patients with the diagnosis of unstable or pre-
infarction angina have been treated with IABP counterpulsation.
The balloon has been successful in relieving pain completely in 39
of these. All patients had coronary arteriography performed while

on IABP support; 38 were operated upon with 36 survivors.

Patients with crescendo angina and widespread electrocardiographic changes suggesting main left coronary artery or severe triple
vessel disease have also been supported through angiography and
operation by the balloon.

Early in our coronary arterial surgical experience, several
patients with main left coronary artery stenosis developed
increasing ischemia, measured by precordial ECG leads and rising
pulmonary capillary wedge presssures upon the induction of
anesthesia for their bypass operation, and we also experienced
severe tachyarrhythmias leading to fibrillation and shock at the
time of cannulation of the right atrium. For this reason, some
patients with main left coronary artery stenosis have had an intra
aortic balloon inserted as the first step in an elective coronary
bypass procedure.

Cardiogenic shock remains the largest indication for IABP
treatment. Experience with these patients has led us to moderate,
somewhat, the protocol initially used in treating cardiogenic shock.
The balloon is still inserted as early as possible after the onset
of shock. The majority of patients will show a salutory response
to this treatment, with improvement in cardiac output, urinary
output, and sensorium, and reduction of the pulmonary capillary
wedge pressure. If there is a concurrent interventricular septal
rupture or mitral regurgitation, diminution of shunt and left
atrial pressure, respectively, can be demonstrated. Alpha-blocking
drugs and pressors in appropriate combinations are sometimes used
in this setting.

If the patient does not significantly improve after the
insertion of the balloon, an inexorable downhill course can be
predicted. Those patients who do improve are tested for "balloon
dependence" after 24 hours.

TABLE II

HEMODYNAMIC CRITERIA FOR "BALLOON DEPENDENCE"

1. Cardiac Index <2 L/min/M^2
2. Mean arterial blood pressure <60 mm Hg.
    Product of #1 x #2 <120
3. Pulmonary capillary wedge pressure >20 mm Hg.
4. Recurrent angina pectoris
5. Recurrent arrhythmias

If their cardiac performance diminishes to a cardiac output of less than 2 L/min/M^2, the mean arterial pressure falls to 60 mm Hg., the pulmonary capillary wedge pressure rises to 20 mm Hg., or there is recurrent angina, "balloon dependence" is established, and the IABP is no longer weaned. The patient is then taken to the catheterization laboratory and cardiac catheterization and coronary and ventricular angiography performed. If the patient is deemed operable by the criteria in Table III, operation is then performed within 24-48 hours. (See Figure 4)

TABLE III

CRITERIA OF OPERABILITY IN CARDIOGENIC SHOCK

Short period of shock

Good response to inotropy or blocking agents

Hemodynamic improvement with IABP

Akinesia involving less than 60% of left ventricle

Distal coronary arteries adequate for bypass

Vascularity of hypokinetic areas of left ventricle
   adjacent to infarction

The balloon therefore is used as both a treatment modality and as a "triage" device to determine which patients will possibly benefit from acute revascularization. Its use has allowed our group to treat 50-60 such patients a year in a moderately calm and comfortable manner without totally disrupting an elective schedule of 1,000 cardiac surgical operations yearly.

The Massachusetts General Hospital has six AVCO IABP consoles; on several occasions it has been necessary to borrow consoles from the other units, for as many as 8 patients have been balloon-pumped simultaneously.

There have been a total of 934 balloon involved procedures. 506 patients have had balloons inserted, 5 twice; 399 patients have had balloon pumps removed and 29 patients have had attempted insertion of intra aortic balloons with no success. The fate of those 29 patients can be seen in Table IV.

FIG. 4   PROTOCOL FOR TREATMENT OF PATIENTS WITH CARDIOGENIC SHOCK

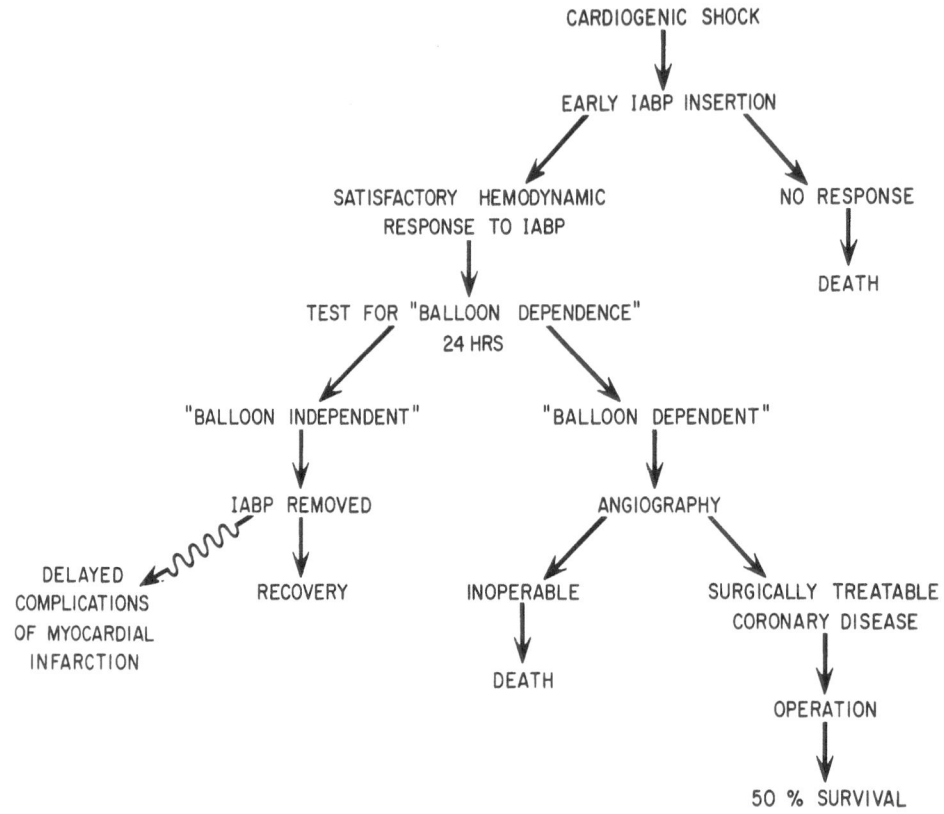

TABLE IV

FATE OF PATIENTS FOLLOWING UNSUCCESSFUL
ATTEMPTS TO INSERT IABP TRANS-FEMORALLY

Unable to insert IABP trans-femorally   29

   No other attempt made
     Survival (pre-operative)   5
     Dead   24

Unable to insert IABP trans-femorally   14

   Inserted in
     Common iliac   5
     Abdominal aorta   2
     Ascending aorta   7

24 patients in whom a balloon could not be inserted died; five patients in whom the attempted balloon insertion was an elective adjunct to a surgical procedure survived operation. 14 patients have had balloon insertions in vessels other than the common femoral artery, after attempts at inserting the device through the peripheral artery were unsuccessful. The most frequent cause of failure has been severe atherosclerosis of the aorta and iliac vessels, although several female patients have had femoral vessels too small to accept even a 20cc. balloon which is mounted on a 12F catheter.

Severe atherosclerosis has contributed also to a series of vascular complications as outlined in Table V.

TABLE V

VASCULAR COMPLICATIONS OF IABP

Ischemic limb requiring
IABP removal   12

  Required amputation   1
  Post-removal claudication 4

Arterial injury requiring
replacement of femoral artery   2

Post-removal thrombosis of
femoral artery   2

Bleeding from oversewn
side-arm graft   1

Perforation of common
iliac artery   2

Dissection of aorta   8

  Asymptomatic   4
  Symptomatic   4
    Renal ischemia   2
    Gangrenous bowel   2

Perforation of the common iliac artery was uniformly fatal, while dissection of the aorta was not. 4 patients with dissections augmented well and the injury was notable only at postoperative coronary arteriography or post mortem examination. The other vascular complications were easily treatable with local procedures as they were identified.

Patients with an indwelling intra-aortic balloon are treated with intravenous Heparin, except postoperatively, and with low-molecular weight Dextran, to help reduce platelet loss. There have been only 8 documented emboli, 17 bleeding episodes directly related to the wound and 3 gastrointestinal hemorrhages which stopped when heparinization was discontinued.

TABLE VI

HEMATOLOGIC COMPLICATIONS OF
IABP COUNTERPULSATIONS

Wound bleeding/hematoma		17
G.I. bleeding (Heparin/Dextran)		3
Emboli		8
Testis	1	
Kidney	2	
Lower extremities	5	

The balloon catheter exits from a groin incision which is treated aseptically in the same fashion as intravenous hyperalimentation catheters, with sterile dressings reapplied aseptically on alternate days. 8 patients have had superficial wound infections requiring local dressing care. 5 patients had febrile episodes associated with positive blood cultures and cultures of the balloon when it was removed. Because of the presence of prosthetic material at the femoral artery insertion site, a three week course of antibiotics has been used. No patient has had a mycotic aneurysm of the femoral arterotomy; all balloon pumps have been removed in either the Surgical Intensive Care, Coronary Care, or Myocardial Infarction Research Units, not in the operating room.

The intra aortic balloon pump, therefore, has become an increasingly frequently and easily used aid in supporting cardiac function in patients suffering from acute myocardial ischemia and those at significant risk to experience further myocardial injury. Its effect is predictable and reproducible and the patient/balloon interface can be managed with few technical problems and a low percentage of surgical complications.

REFERENCES

1. Buckley, M.J., Mundth, E.D., Daggett, W.M., DeSanctis, R.W., Sanders, C.A. and Austen, W.G.: Surgical therapy for early complications of myocardial infarction. Surgery, 70:814, 1971.

2. Mundth, E.D., Buckley, M.J., Daggett, W.M., Sanders, C.A. and Austen, W.G.: Surgery for complications of acute myocardial infarction. Circulation, 45:1279, 1972.

3. Kantrowitz, A. and Kantrowitz, A.: Experimental augmentation of coronary flow be retardation of arterial pressure pulse. Surgery, 34:678, 1953.

4. Clauss, R.H., Birtwell, W.C., Albertal, G., Lunzar, S., Taylor, W.J., Fosberg, A.M. and Harken, D.E.: Assisted circulation, I. The arterial counterpulsation. Journal of Thoracic and Cardiovascular Surgery, 41:447, 1961.

5. Moulopoulos, S.D., Topaz, S. and Kolff, W.J.: Diastolic balloon pumping (with carbon dioxide) in the aorta - a mechanical assistance to the failing circulation. American Heart Journal, 63:669, 1962.

6. Weber, K.T., Janecki, J.S. and Walker, A.A.: Intra aortic balloon pumping: An analysis of several variables affecting balloon performance. Transactions of the American Society of Artificial Internal Organs, 18:486, 1972.

7. Powell, W.J., Jr., Daggett, W.M., Magro, A.E., Bianco, J.A., Buckley, M.J., Sanders, C.A., Kantrowitz, A.R. and Austen, W.G.: Effects of intra aortic balloon counterpulsation on cardiac performance, oxygen consumption and coronary blood flow in dogs. Circulation Research, 26:753, 1970.

8. Maroko, P.R., Bernstein, E.F., Libby, P., DeLaria, G.A., Covell, J.W., Ross, J., Jr. and Braunwald, E.: Effects of intra aortic balloon counterpulsation on the severity of myocardial ischemic injury following acute coronary occlusion. Circulation, 45: 1150, 1972.

9. Kantrowitz, A., Tjønnelund, S., Krakauer, J.S., Phillips, S.J., Freed, P.S. and Butner, A.N.: Mechanical intra aortic cardiac assistance in cardiogenic shock. Archives of Surgery, 97: 1000, 1968.

10. Buckley, M.J., Leinbach, R.C., Kastor, J.A., Laird, J.D.,
     Kantrowitz, A.R., Madras, P.N., Sanders, C.A. and Austen, W.G.:
     Hemodynamic evaluation of intra aortic balloon pumping in man.
     Circulation, 41(Suppl. II):130, 1970.

11. Page, D.L., Caulfield, J.B., Kastor, J.A., DeSanctis, R.W.
     and Sanders, C.A.: Myocardial changes associated with
     cardiogenic shock. New England Journal of Medicine, 285:
     133, 1971.

12. Hershberg, P.I. and Kaplan, E.M.: Circulatory support in acute
     myocardial infarction. Advances in Cardiology, 6:173, 1971.

13. Dunkman, W.B., Leinbach, R.C., Buckley, M.J., Mundth, E.D.,
     Kantrowitz, A.R., Austen, W.G. and Sanders, C.A.: Clinical
     and hemodynamic results of intra aortic balloon pumping and
     surgery in cardiogenic shock. Circulation, 46:465, 1972.

14. Mundth, E.D., Yurchak, P.M., Buckley, M.J., Leinbach, R.C.,
     Kantrowitz, A. and Austen, W.G.: Circulatory assistance and
     emergency direct coronary artery surgery for shock complicating
     acute myocardial infarction. New England Journal of Medicine,
     283:1382, 1970.

15. Buckley, M.J., Craver, J.M., Gold, H.K., Mundth, E.D., Daggett,
     W.M. and Austen, W.G.: Intra aortic balloon pump assist for
     cardiogenic shock after cardiopulmonary bypass. Circulation,
     47(Suppl. III):90, 1973.

16. Buckberg, G.D., Towers, B., Paglia, D.E., Mulder, D.G. and
     Maloney, J.V.: Subendocardial ischemia after cardiopulmonary
     bypass. Journal of Thoracic and Cardiovascular Surgery, 64:
     669, 1972.

17. Philips, P.A., Marty, A.T. and Myamoto, A.M.: A clinical
     method for detecting subendocardial ischemia following
     cardiopulmonary bypass. Presented at the 54th meeting of
     The American Association for Thoracic Surgery, Las Vegas,
     Nevada, April, 1974.

18. Buckberg, G.D., Fixler, D.E., Archie, J.P. and Hoffman, J.I.E.:
     Experimental subendocardial ischemia in dogs with normal
     coronary arteries. Circulation Research, 30:67, 1972.

DISCUSSION

CHAIRMAN: MR. D. WATSON

JACKSON: I wonder if you could possibly confirm what you said
about your criteria for angiography when you have a patient who
is in cardiogenic shock who is established on the balloon? Do
I understand you to say that if the patient becomes balloon
independent then the treatment is just to take the balloon out
and perform interval surgery as necessary?
McENANY: Yes, that is right. The first slide showed that the
people who become balloon independent have a 50% mortality at
six months. What we generally do is interval coronary arteriography at the end of a month and if they have what we consider
to be life threatening multiple vessel disease or left main artery
disease, then we operate within the next week or so. But this
group, the ones that survive decannulation, do have a 50% mortality
at six months. The thing that has changed so much in the last two
years is the frenetic pace that we used to work at. Instead of
rushing from ballooning to arteriography to operation, we now
determine balloon dependence or independence and put the patients
on a schedule for more leisurely investigation and treatment as
necessary. Nothing is done at two or three in the morning any
more.
HOLLINRAKE: In patients who have shock following an infarct, who
become balloon dependent, do you go on to operate on those after
performing coronary arteriography?
McENANY: Yes we do. As of July 1st, 1975 we have now 61 patients
in cardiogenic shock, balloon dependent and "surgically treatable."
Of those three had VSD's closed and three had mitral valves
replaced. 31 have survived to leave hospital alive, so we have a
50% immediate survival. But most patients who are balloon
dependent are not "surgically treatable." We no longer think that

surgical treatment of cardiogenic shock is desperate last ditch therapy. If you take the patients with demonstrable improvement on the balloon, implying that they have at least 50% of their ventricle still able to function, we believe that thanks to this treatment 50% of them will be alive in one year - this is opposed to certain death if not treated with the balloon. We do not think this is desperate therapy.

HOLLINRAKE: The implication is that you are concentrating on the viable muscle rather than trying to revascularise any muscle that has been infarcted.

McENANY: You cannot make necrotic muscle work. If the patient has had a massive anteroseptal infarction, the front of the ventricle is akinetic and the anterior descending artery does not show up on the arteriogram, we do not graft that type of patient any more because all you get is a haemorrhagic infarct and that makes things worse. We try to revascularise peri-infarction tissue not necrotic ischaemic tissue.

MOORE: What proportion of your patients have a Swan-Ganz catheter put in?

McENANY: Everyone who comes through the coronary care unit has had a Swan-Ganz catheter put in. People who have the balloon put in in the operating room generally have a left atrial catheter but all the others have a Swan-Ganz. There are frequently 15 or 20 such catheters in use in our hospital at any one time.

DEVERALL: Do you have a cardiac output monitor and does it work?

McENANY: We measure the cardiac output by two methods. For many years we have been wedded to the green dye. Now I.L. (Instrumentation Laboratories) in Massachusetts have produced a very good thermal dilution probe which are, in fact, thermistors inside a Swan-Ganz catheter. We are at present happy with the I.L. equipment.

DEVERALL: What is that little console that sits on top of the AVCO system?

McENANY: That little console is a Medtronic square-wave coupled pulse generator which we use for sequential atrial and ventricular pacing.

MONRO: Have any of your patients been children?

McENANY: We have not inserted a balloon into a child although we have been on the point of it once or twice.

MONRO: Do you know of anyone who has? I know that AVCO are the only people that have brought out paediatric catheters.

McENANY: Yes, there are two: one is a 12cc balloon on a 10 French catheter and the other is a 7cc balloon on an 8 French catheter.

DEVERALL: We successfully pumped a six year old. The only problem was getting it in. The femoral artery transected in the process but we managed to retrieve the situation. The clinical details were rather difficult. It was a child with Fallot's tetralogy who had for a reason I do not understand, massive biventricular hypertrophy who developed a low cardiac output

after operation. We attributed this to subendocardial damage,
etc., etc. There was no doubt that diastolic augmentation changed
the whole clinical course of that child. It was almost as if
we had turned a switch on and completely supported all you
suggested would happen.

MACARTNEY: The interesting thing is that you said you would not
use it in a patient who developed late cardiogenic shock after
operation.

McENANY: Let me put it this way. We have an overall 9% mortality
rate in our unit. Some of these 9% are people who leave the
operating room on a little bit of Dopamine or a little bit of
adrenaline, and they get worse over the next four days or so.
People like that do not respond satisfactorily to balloon
pumping. I think that unless there is an identifiable insult
such as myocardial infarction or intraoperative subendocardial
ischaemia then balloon pumping is not worthwhile.

MACARTNEY: But the patient who gets in to trouble within the
first 24 hours, you would consider pumping?

McENANY: We do that. In fact we sometimes insert the balloon
at the end of the operation.

MEARNS: You suggest you have sequential pacing available. Have
you seen any effect of balloon pumping in these patients who have
heart block with their infarct?

McENANY: We use pacing as an inotropic agent. We pace rather
than use pressors. There is a significant number of patients we
operate on for acute ischaemia in shock who have junctional
rhythms and who develop shock after their operation for a finite
time. Pacing has been impressively life-saving in that group of
patients. Pacing is also extremely satisfactory in post-operative
patients because you can run the balloon off the pacemaker. This
allows the surgeon to use electrocautery. The other thing you
can do is run the balloon off the pulmonary artery pacing.

MEARNS: I was thinking of the acute situation of cardiogenic
shock.

McENANY: As a surgeon I do not have an awful lot of experience
with transvenous pacing. Once they have gone into the operating
room we put on epicardial atrio-ventricular pacing wires.

JACKSON: I was just going to add a comment, if I might to that
question of pacing function, block and the question of sequential
pacing. We, in fact, have got 30 patients whom we have ballooned
in shock and two of whom have been in block. We have been
successful with Douglas Chamberlain's University of Sussex
pacemaker which is basically synchronous rather than sequential.
He has demonstrated 50% improvements in output in shocked patients
just by putting them on sequential pacing even if their idio-
ventricular rate is reasonable because of the contribution of
atrial transport.

McENANY: That is our experience too.

CHAIRMAN: We must come to an end there. Most of us have patients

who have benefitted from balloon pumping and we are most grateful
to Dr. McEnany for giving us the current thinking on this subject
at the Massachusetts General Hospital.

As this is the last contribution to this conference I feel I must
thank the organisers for giving us such an interesting two days.